Eating for

Sustained Energy 2

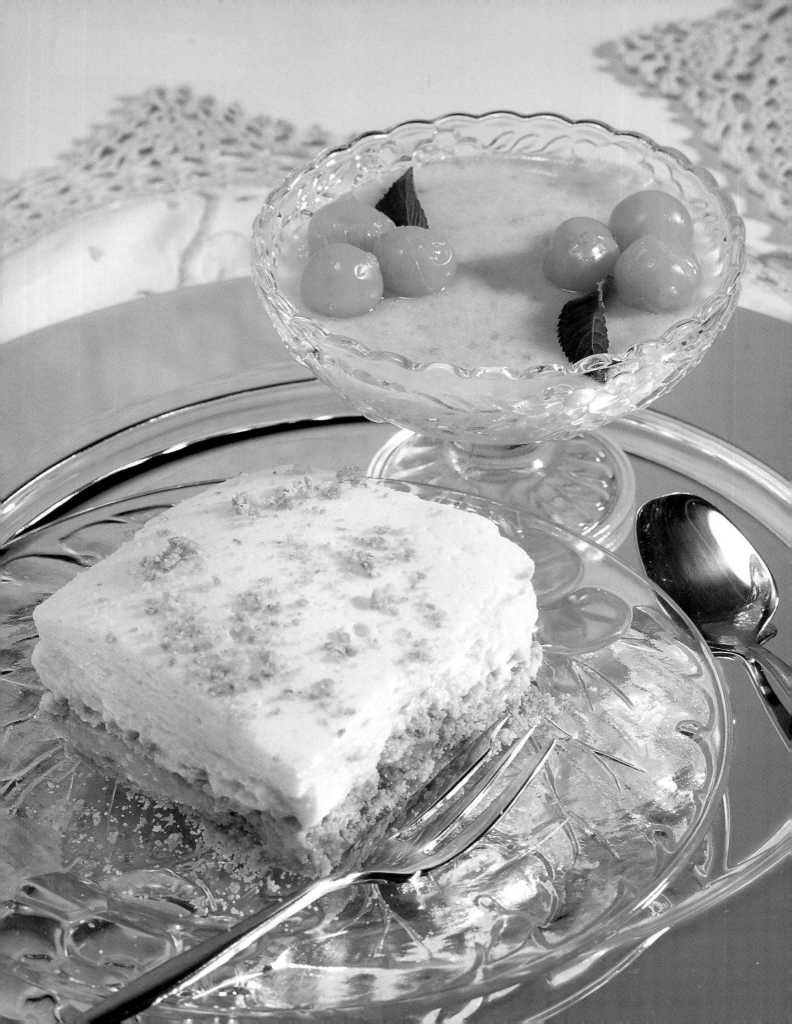

Eating for
Sustained
Energy 2

Gabi Steenkamp RD(SA) and Liesbet Delport RD(SA)

To all diabetics, who for so long have had to eat 'special' foods containing no sugar, that often tasted like cardboard. Thanks to the Glycaemic Index, they can now enjoy the normal, lower fat, lower GI foods that are best for everyone who wishes to enjoy sustained energy.

First published in 2004 by Tafelberg
40 Heerengracht, Cape Town

10 9 8 7 6 5 4 3 2 1

PUBLISHER	Anita Pyke
EDITOR	Pat Barton
PHOTOGRAPHY	Willie van Heerden
FOOD STYLIST	Engela van Eyssen
COVER PHOTOGRAPH	Neville Lockhart
STYLING	Wilma Howells
DESIGN AND TYPESETTING	Lindie Metz
REPRODUCTION	Unifoto (Pty) Ltd, Cape Town
Printing	Tien Wah Press (Pte) Ltd, Singapore
ISBN	0 624041 25 5

Contents

Foreword   7

Introduction   8

   How the Glycaemic Index (GI) is determined   9

   The Glycaemic load (GL)   10

   How to make the Glycaemic Index (GI) work for you   12

   Healthy eating   12

   Conditions that benefit from the lower GI, lower fat way of eating   14

      Diabetes melitus   14

      Hypoglycaemia (low blood sugar)   15

      Coronary Heart Disease (CHD)   16

      Attention Deficit Hyperactivity Disorder (ADHD)

       or Attention Deficit Disorder (ADD)   17

   Weight management   18

   Sports nutrition   19

   The vegetarian diet   19

   Nutritional analysis of recipes   20

The Glycaemic Index List of South African Lower Fat Foods   22

Recipes

   Breakfasts   24

   Soups   30

   Salads   34

   Light Meals   38

   Chicken dishes   48

   Fish dishes   58

   Vegetables and vegetarian dishes   64

   Meat dishes   78

   Desserts   86

   Cakes, breads, biscuits and rusks   96

   Basics   120

   Drinks   122

Recommended food/product list   124

Index   126

Acknowledgements   128

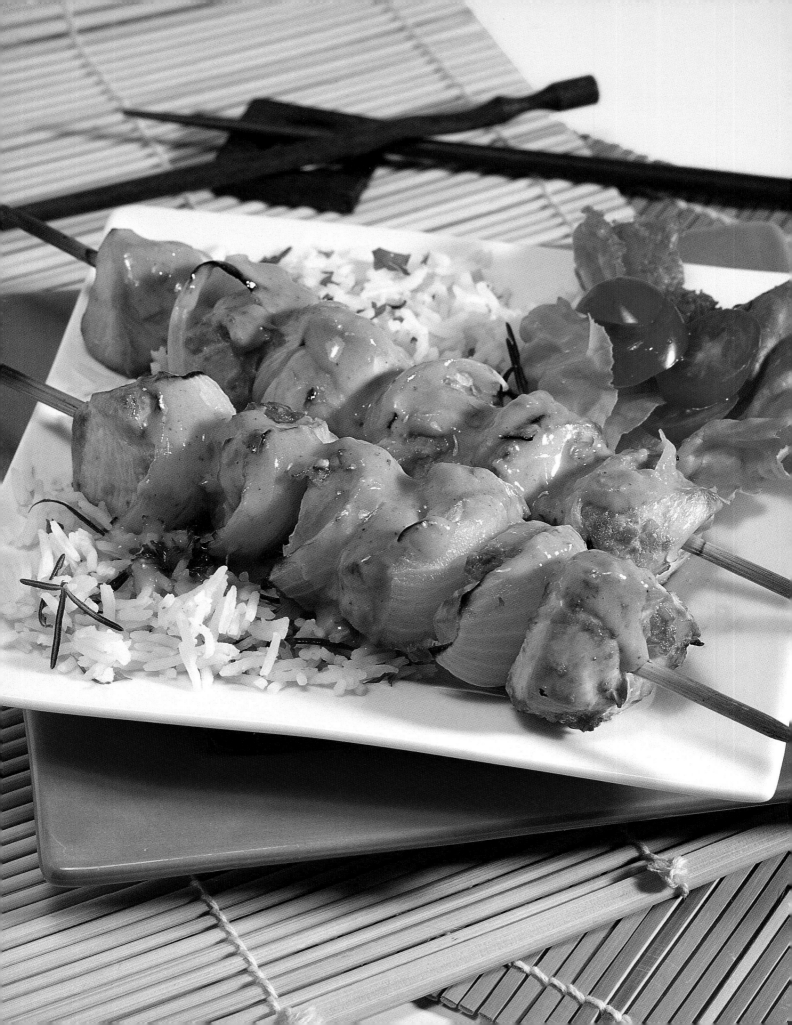

Foreword

When we originally put together *Eating for Sustained Energy*, we had several aims: we wanted each recipe to be really tasty, quick and easy to make, using ingredients that are affordable and readily available in any home, while also being lower in fat and having lower GI values than regular recipes. Our readers assure us just about every day that we have reached each and every one of these aims. In fact, we have had so many requests for more recipes from satisfied readers that we decided to compile *Eating for Sustained Energy 2*. And so, after many hours of hard work and experimenting … here it is!

Like its predecessor there is, once again, a photograph for each recipe, so that you can see clearly what you're going to make and what the end product will look like. Some of our readers tell us that it's just as well we have provided a photograph for each recipe, because if they had had to judge solely by the list of ingredients, many of the recipes – especially in the baking section – would have seemed to be for muesli!

When we started out writing the first *Eating for Sustained Energy*, we did not have a publisher and we had no idea that recipes of this type would be so popular. What we did have was plenty of enthusiasm as well as the knowledge that it's not that difficult to compile tasty, healthy recipes; in fact, both of us were cooking and baking dishes like these for our families every day! And we felt they should to be shared with you, the public.

More than 30 000 copies of *Eating for Sustained Energy* have been sold in the three years the book has been on the market, and it continues to sell well, so we know that these recipes really work. Used regularly, they help to lower diabetics' blood glucose from high levels – such as 20 mmol/l, sometimes, to below 10 mmol/l – and reduce cholesterol levels, blood pressure, hyperinsulinaemia and insulin resistance, as well as alleviating the symptoms of chronic candida, polycystic ovarian syndrome (PCOS) and inflammatory diseases such as arthritis. They also help children who suffer from Attention Deficit (Hyperactivity) Disorder (AD[H]D) to concentrate better, overweight people to lose weight more easily, fatigued people to have more energy and sportsmen to perform better.

In *Eating for Sustained Energy 2*, we have included a new value in the nutritional information box, the Glycaemic load (GL). This is explained in detail, in easy-to-understand terms, in the introduction. We have also condensed the introduction; should you require more detail, please see the introduction to the first *Eating for Sustained Energy* or visit the website of the GI Foundation of SA (GIFSA) at www.gifoundation.com.

Our very own *South African Glycaemic Index Guide* has also been of great help to many. The first printing has sold out and the new, updated version, including all the GI values of foods that were tested during the past year, has a new, more modern 'jacket'. Many people like to keep the GI Guide with them when they shop, so that they can quickly check the GI of any food.

Our book on weight maintenance, *Eat Smart and Stay Slim: the GI Diet*, is rapidly carving a niche for itself among the plethora of slimming books. People say that it helps them to get their mind right about getting thin and staying thin. The book contains so much information that they want to read it over and over again until they feel they have mastered the contents. In addition, it makes such compelling reading that they cannot put it down once they've started reading it. This book contains a few recipes at the back (some of which are also all included in this recipe book), as well as a handy section that details meals for a week, which will help you lose weight by combining any breakfast, lunch and dinner, as well as two to three snacks per day. Other invaluable information – such as how to get out of the compulsive eating habit, how to read food labels, and how to fat-proof your meals – is provided, as well as the motivation to start exercising regularly.

Eating For Sustained Energy 2 provides many more recipes, all of them delicious, which will help to manage weight, control blood glucose levels, ensure healthy eating in general, and improve sports performance.

May you enjoy this book as much as you did all the others!

Introduction

Most people feel they could do with more sustained energy.

'I'm always tired!'

'I have no energy!'

We hear comments like these every day in our modern, stressed world, where chronic fatigue is the norm.

We believe that most of the solution to the problem lies in eating correctly. By learning how to use the Glycaemic Index (GI) and consuming a lower fat diet, one can attain an endless supply of energy. Resorting to all sorts of 'pick-me-up' tonics or caffeine, alcohol or cigarettes to relax will no longer be necessary. Carbohydrate is the body's source of fuel and, if you consume the right type at the right time, the result should be sustained energy, instead of highs and lows – feeling hyped up one moment, and depressed the next. Eating the lower fat way and following the Glycaemic Index (GI) will regulate blood glucose levels, keeping them stable, and result in your feeling great all the time.

In the past, it was assumed that complex carbohydrates or starches, such as potatoes, mealie meal and bread, were digested and absorbed slowly, resulting in only a slight rise in blood glucose levels. Simple sugars, on the other hand, were believed to be digested and absorbed quickly, producing a large and rapid rise in blood glucose levels. We now know that these assumptions were incorrect, and that nobody, including diabetics, now needs to avoid sugar altogether, provided that they use it correctly. In fact, we know that ordinary sugar has a slightly more favourable effect on the blood glucose levels of normal and diabetic individuals than potatoes, bread and a few other starches do, if used on their own.

As early as the 1930s, scientists challenged the traditionally held view that the metabolic effects of carbohydrates (CHO) could be predicted by classifying them as either 'simple' or 'complex'. In the 1970s, researchers such as Otto and Crapo examined the glycaemic impact of a range of foods containing carbohydrate. To standardise the interpretation of glycaemic response (the effect of food on blood glucose levels) data, Jenkins and others at the University of Toronto, Canada, proposed the Glycaemic Index (GI) in 1981.

The **Glycaemic Index (GI)** is a rating of foods according to their actual effect on blood glucose levels. Jenkins' work disproved the assumption that equivalent quantities of CHO from different foods cause similar glycaemic responses. Furthermore, the researchers concluded that the CHO exchange lists that have for years been used to regulate the eating plans of most diabetics, do not reflect the physiological effects of foods and are therefore no longer adequate to control blood glucose levels. In studies conducted over the past two decades, scientists have shown that it is not so much the quantity of carbohydrate, but rather **its rate of digestion and absorption into the bloodstream**, that determines the physiological response of the body. Worldwide research conducted since then confirms that the new way of ranking foods according to their actual effect on blood glucose is scientifically more correct.

The Glycaemic Index (GI) was developed as a result. The index **ranks foods on a scale of 0–100, according to their actual effect on blood glucose levels**. In South Africa – and, indeed, most of the world – glucose is taken as 100, since it causes the greatest and most rapid rise in blood glucose levels, and all other foods are rated in comparison to glucose. It must, however, be noted that some Glycaemic Index testing has been published using bread as the reference food; while this is completely acceptable in the scientific world, it could create the impression that some GI values from different sources seem to differ. So when you are checking GI values, always establish first whether the reference food used is glucose or bread. The *SA Glycaemic Index Guide* (available from the Glycaemic Index Foundation of SA [www.gifoundation.com], your dietician, local bookstore, health shop or pharmacy) is one of the most reliable sources of GI values of foods commonly eaten in South Africa. All the values published in the guide are based on glucose as the reference food, and it contains the most recent GI values of foods tested in SA and internationally. Since the Glycaemic Index is a ranking of foods based on their actual effect on blood glucose levels, instead of on assumptions, it is a much more accurate tool to use in the regulation of blood glucose levels.

Using the GI concept, **persons with diabetes** and those suffering from other blood glucose control problems – low blood sugar levels i.e. **hypoglycaemia, ME (chronic fatigue syndrome), hyperinsulinaemia and insulin resistance, polycystic ovarian syndrome (PCOS), candidiasis, inflammatory diseases (such as arthritis), fibromyalgia syndrome (FMS), and Attention Deficit (Hyperactivity) Disorder (AD[H]D)**, in children – as well as **sportsmen**, can all optimise their blood glucose control.

Serum triglycerides, LDL cholesterol levels, total cholesterol and **high blood pressure levels** can be lowered if the GI concept is used in combination with lower fat eating, and HDL cholesterol (the 'good' cholesterol) levels may be increased. For those who want to lose weight, the increased satiety value of a lower GI diet and the fact that less insulin (a fat storer) is secreted, result in greater fat loss. For a comprehensive, easy-to-understand weight management book based on these principles, see *Eat Smart and Stay Slim: the GI Diet*.

Even people suffering from **cancer, gout** and **irritable bowel syndrome (IBS)** can benefit from lower fat eating and the GI concept, although they should consult a dietician as some other adjustments will have to be made to their diets (see www.gifoundation.com for a list of dieticians who use the GI concept). Foods that have a low GI value release glucose slowly and steadily into the bloodstream and do not over-stimulate insulin secretion. High insulin levels are implicated in many diseases engendered by our modern lifestyle: high blood pressure, for instance, as well as high cholesterol levels, high triglyceride levels, diabetes, hypoglycaemia, obesity, polycystic ovarian syndrome (PCOS) and coronary heart disease.

Apart from being lower GI, all the recipes in this book are also **lower in fat**. Fat, especially saturated fat, is the main dietary cause of heart disease and high cholesterol levels, being overweight, hyperinsulinaemia and insulin resistance, cancer, high blood pressure and gout. In addition, irritable bowel syndrome (IBS) is aggravated by a high fat intake, and saturated fat is the main dietary promoter of cancer. High fat intakes also result in the body's insulin working less effectively, which may play a role in the development of reactive hypoglycaemia and, eventually, diabetes. Furthermore, it was found that it is fat and not really carbohydrates (starches, vegetables, fruit and sugars) that are fattening. It requires no effort for the body to turn dietary fat into body fat, whereas it takes a lot of effort and energy to convert carbohydrates and protein into body fat, although it is easier for the body to turn high GI carbohydrates into body fat, due to the over-secretion of insulin. Most thin people consume a lower fat diet that's high in carbohydrates and moderate in protein. Fat people follow high-fat diets, which are usually high GI as well. Not more than 30% of the total energy value in our diet should come from fat. In this book, we have heeded that recommendation and the fat content of every meal serving is kept as close to 10g of fat (or below) as possible. If you would like more detailed information about the quantity and type of fat per portion and per day, consult our weight management book, *Eat Smart and Stay Slim: The GI Diet*, and consult a dietician, who can then advise and support you as you walk the path of weight management.

How the Glycaemic Index (GI) is determined

The blood glucose response (BGR) to glucose (reference food) of at least 8–12 people per food tested, is measured. This is done on three different occasions for every person, and the average value is the BGR for that person. The blood glucose response to glucose is given the value of 100. Of all foods, glucose is absorbed most quickly and generally causes the greatest and most rapid rise in blood glucose level. Blood glucose responses of all other carbohydrate foods are also measured by actual blood tests in the same 8–12 people per food tested, and rated in comparison to glucose for that specific person. The average GI of the food for the group is allocated the GI value that can be applied to the general population. One could say that the GI of a food represents its ability to raise blood glucose levels.

Often, the GI of a given food is not what one would expect. For example, the GI of South African brown bread is 81, whereas the average GI of sweetened low-fat fruit yoghurt is only 33. For this reason, all foods that contain carbohydrate need to be tested in order to determine their GI. One could be very far out if one guessed the GI value of a food. The GI of more than 800 foods has been determined worldwide and more foods are being tested on a weekly basis, overseas as well as in South Africa. For a complete reference guide to the Glycaemic Index of foods commonly used in South Africa, see *The South African Glycaemic Index Guide*.

FACTORS THAT INFLUENCE THE GLYCAEMIC INDEX (GI)

Ongoing studies reveal that the body's responses to food are much more complex than was originally appreciated. The following factors have an influence on the digestion and absorption of carbohydrates, and thus on how foods affect blood glucose levels. In other words, these factors affect the Glycaemic Index of the food, which is the measure, on a numerical scale, of how carbohydrate-containing foods affect blood sugar levels.

THE DEGREE OF STARCH GELATINISATION Gelatinisation of starches occurs when the starchy food is exposed to liquid and/or heat (i.e. cooking). When potatoes are boiled, the heat and water expand the hard compact granules (which usually make raw potatoes difficult to digest) into swollen granules. Some granules even burst and free the individual starch molecules, which means they are easier to digest. (Remember that starch is a string of glucose molecules.) The same happens when a sauce is thickened with flour or cornflour. The water binds with the starch in the presence of heat and gelatinises the flour, making it easier to digest. For this reason, many confectionery items that contain sugar have a lower GI than those without! The sugar binds with the water, preventing it from binding with the flour, and thereby limiting gelatinisation. The less a starch is gelatinised, the slower it is digested and absorbed. In other words, it will have a lower GI.

PARTICLE SIZE Intact grains such as whole-wheat, whole corn, whole rye, whole oats (groats) and whole barley have much lower GI values than flours made from the same grains, because they take longer to digest.

PROCESSING Milling, beating, liquidising, grinding, mixing, mashing and refining foods raises the GI of that food by making it more easily available to the body. For this reason, we restrict beating and liquidising as preparation and cooking methods in the recipes.

THE CHEMICAL COMPOSITION OF THE STARCH Starches, such as rice, can have different types of starch structures that affect their digestibility. Some types of rice, such as basmati and Tastic rice, have a higher amylose content. Amylose is made up of long straight chains of glucose molecules packed closely together, and therefore more difficult to digest. Other kinds of rice have a higher amylopectin content – branched chains of glucose molecules that do not pack closely together, are less dense, much easier to digest and thus have a higher GI. Rice that contains predominantly amylose (e.g. Tastic white rice) is inclined to be loose when cooked, whereas rice that contains predominantly amylopectin is inclined to be more sticky when cooked (e.g. arborio, risotto rice).

FIBRE: TYPE AND CONTENT Foods containing soluble fibre – such as oat bran, less processed oats, legumes (beans, peas and lentils), citrus and deciduous fruits – have a lowering effect on the GI, because they delay gastric emptying. Insoluble fibre such as that found in digestive bran, has very little effect on the digestibility of the carbohydrate foods in which it is found. So, foods containing wheat (digestive) bran do not have a lower GI than foods that do not contain the bran, unless they contain digestive bran in large quantities, e.g. in high-fibre cereal. Brown bread and white bread have similar GI values, and so do refined and unrefined mealie meal.

SUGAR Sugar may lower the GI of foods that have a very high GI, because sugar has a lower GI than many starches, and also because it competes with the starch for the liquid for gelatinisation in baking.

A good example of this is Rice Krispies that have a high GI. When they are sugar-coated, the GI is lower, so Strawberry Pops have a lower GI than Rice Krispies! But this does not mean that one is better than the other. Likewise, sugar-free Weet-Bix has a higher GI than regular Weet-Bix, which contains sugar. As mentioned above, sugar can also lower the GI of baked goods, since it is inclined to bind with the fluid in baking, preventing it from binding with the flour and thereby limiting gelatinisation.

PROTEIN AND FAT The presence of protein and fat in food may lower the GI because of the interaction of these nutrients with each other and with carbohydrate, and because both protein and fat slow down the rate at which food leaves the stomach. It's not advisable to eat too much protein or fat, however. Protein tends to wear out the body's insulin; and fat intake results in a decrease of the effectiveness of insulin. Protein also overtaxes the kidneys and over-consumption can lead to osteoporosis, arthritis and gout.

ANTI-NUTRIENTS Phytates, lectins and polyphenols (tannins) usually slow digestion and decrease the GI. They are ordinary constituents of many vegetables, legumes, fruit and bran.

ACIDITY The more acid a food is, the lower the GI of that food. Naturally fermented sorghum porridge, for example, has a higher GI than cooked sorghum porridge, to which an acid such as vinegar or lemon juice has been added. Fruits that are more tart in flavour also have lower GI values, and sourdough breads, e.g. sourdough rye bread, have a lower GI value as well.

COOKING, which increases the digestibility of the food, usually has the effect of raising the GI of that food.

RESISTANT STARCH, which develops in some cooked and cooled-down starches, and vegetables and fruit, has a slight lowering effect on the GI, especially in the case of mealie meal and samp. So cold cooked maize porridge (mealie-meal porridge) has a lower GI than the hot, freshly prepared porridge, because the body has difficulty in digesting the resistant starch that develops when some cooked starches are cooled down.

SPEED OF EATING Studies have shown that blood glucose levels rise less rapidly when foods are eaten more slowly.

The Glycaemic load (GL)

A new concept, called the Glycaemic load (GL), which was developed by scientists from Harvard University, USA, 'fine tunes' the Glycaemic Index (GI) concept. It addresses concerns about rating carbohydrate foods as either 'good' or 'bad' on the basis of their GI. There is no such thing as a good or bad carbohydrate food. All carbohydrate foods can fit into a healthy diet – it all depends on when you eat it, how much you eat, and with what you combine it. For example, although low GI food is usually the preferred choice, a high GI sports drink is perfect during and after running a marathon, as a low GI drink during or after intense exercise could, in fact, can result in hypoglycaemia and insufficient replenishment of glycogen in the muscle and liver.

The Glycaemic load (GL) of a specific food portion is an expression of how much impact ('oomph'), or power the food will have in affecting blood glucose levels. **It is calculated by taking the percentage of the food's carbohydrate content per portion and multiplying it by its Glycaemic Index value**

$$GL = \frac{CHO \text{ content per portion} \times GI}{100}$$

It is thus a measure that incorporates both the quantity and quality of the dietary carbohydrates consumed. Some fruits and vegetables, for example, have higher GI values and might be perceived as 'bad'. Considering the quantity of carbohydrate per portion, however, the GL is low. This means that their effect on blood glucose levels would be minimal. Let us consider a few examples:

- The GI of watermelon is high (GI = 72), but its Glycaemic load is relatively low (GL = 7), because the quantity of carbohydrate in a serving of watermelon (150 g or a 5 cm thick slice) is minimal, as it contains a lot of water. This does not hold true for watermelon juice, however, as the quantity of carbohydrate in a cup of watermelon juice (250 ml) is much higher, and fruit juice is therefore a more concentrated source of carbohydrate.
- The GI of apples is 38 and the GL of 1 medium apple is 5. This means that eating 1 apple will have hardly any effect on blood glucose levels. If you eat an entire 500 g packet of dried apples, however, its GL would be 50, which means that it could have a huge effect on your blood glucose levels, despite its being low GI. This brings us back to the old principle that there is no licence to over-indulge in 'good' or 'bad' foods. But should you indulge in watermelon, it will have an even greater effect on blood glucose levels, due to its high GI value!
- The GI of SA brown bread is high (GI = 81) and the GL of 2 slices (2 x 40 g slices of bread contain 20 g carbohydrate each) is also high (GL = 32), because the quantity of carbohydrate in a hand-cut slice of bread is substantial.

This means that a sandwich made with 2 slices of brown bread will have a marked effect on blood glucose levels as the bread will have an 'oomph' of 32. On the other hand, if you use a thin slice of bread (30 g bread containing 15 g carbohydrate) as part of a mixed meal containing low GI baked beans, ham and salad vegetables, the GL of the meal will be lower and more acceptable (GL = 22). Note that the 2 slices of bread on their own have a higher GL than an entire meal, in which only 1 thin slice of bread is used in combination with other low GI foods.

- The GL of 1 slice of seed loaf is only 8. In contrast to this, a single hand-cut slice of brown or white bread has a GL of 16. This means that ordinary brown or white bread will spike blood glucose levels (higher GL), and the seed loaf will not (lower GL), but this still doesn't mean that you can over-indulge in seed loaf. Fortunately, seed loaf is more filling and it is not as easy to over-indulge in this bread as it is to over-indulge in brown or white bread.
- In addition, the GL of a roll (equivalent to 2 slices of bread) is more than 20, and that of a bagel (equivalent to 3 slices of bread) is more than 30. Imagine what this does to blood glucose levels, as the GI is also high!
- From this we can see that it is quite acceptable to include small quantities of high GI foods in a meal, as long as the bulk of the meal contains lower GI carbohydrate foods (vegetables, fruit, low GI starches, legumes and/or dairy).

New evidence associates high GL meals with an increased risk of heart disease and diabetes, especially in overweight and insulin-resistant people. Therefore, it is advisable to restrict the GL of a typical meal to between 20 and 25 as far as possible, but definitely to keep it below 30. The GL of a typical snack should preferably be between 10 and 15, but if your meals are all close to 30, the total of your snacks should be no more than 10.

This means that you would have to eat fruit for snacks, in order to keep your total daily GL below 100, as the GL of fruit is usually below 10.

What does it mean when a food has a low Glycaemic load (GL)?

A carbohydrate food that has a low Glycaemic load (GL) will have a small impact on blood glucose levels, as it is either not high in carbohydrate and/or has a low Glycaemic Index (GI), so one would have to eat quite a lot of it before it will have any effect on blood glucose levels. In other words, eating any one of the muffins contained in this lower GI, lower fat recipe book, or in *Eating for Sustained Energy 1*, should not raise blood glucose levels significantly, as they have a lower GL.

Having a LOW GL AND A LOW GI is doubly beneficial. A food with a low GI and very little 'push' or 'power' (GL) behind it, will naturally have a very small impact on blood glucose levels, such as low GI vegetables (tomatoes, lettuce, cucumber, onions, asparagus, mushrooms, etc). It follows then that these foods are also not very effective at lowering the GI of high GI foods such as white or brown bread.

Remember: The GI indicates the extent to which a food will raise blood glucose levels, whereas the GL is the 'power' or 'push' behind the GI.

HIGH GI AND HIGH GL means trouble – blood glucose levels will shoot up. This means the food in question will have a lot of 'power' behind the already high GI, and even a small portion will have a marked effect.

Examples of this are cooked mealie meal and potatoes and the regular SA bread mentioned above. These foods are high in carbohydrates and therefore a small portion already contains a lot of carbohydrate. In addition they have high GI values, which aggravates the effect on blood glucose levels.

LOW GI COMBINED WITH A HIGH GL will also impact on blood glucose levels. Remember that the GL is based on the quantity of carbohydrate in a food, and represents the GI in portion size. So the more carbohydrate there is in a food, the higher its GL, i.e. the more 'power' or 'push' behind the GI.

So even low GI foods, if eaten in large quantities, can affect blood glucose levels quite significantly, especially if they are concentrated sources of carbohydrates, e.g. most cakes, dried fruit and dried fruit bars, fruit juices, crisps, chocolates, etc. Crisps and chocolates are also high in fat and/or saturated fat, making them undesirable.

And lastly, a HIGH GI FOOD WITH A LOW GL will not necessarily affect blood glucose levels significantly. A good example here are the high GI vegetables (carrots, pumpkin, etc). They contain only a little carbohydrate and, therefore, in normal portion sizes, will not impact on blood glucose levels even though they have a high GI, as there is not enough 'power' behind the high GI. The proviso is, though, that they are not eaten with other high GI or GL foods.

Please note that the Glycaemic load (GL) of the starch component of most of our low GI breakfasts (such as those in all our lower GI, lower fat recipe books) is about 15, the GL of the starch component of most low GI light meals in our recipe books is between 15 and 20, and the GL of most low GI main meals is about 20.

This means that three meals per day should add up to a GL of between 55 and 70, as most people will add salad and/or fruit to breakfasts and light meals, which also contribute to the GL. This leaves 30–45 GL points for snacks and drinks, as most of these have a GL of 10–15, except for fruit, which has a GL of below 10.

The aim is to keep the total GL per day under 100.

How to make the Glycaemic Index work for you

All foods that have a **GI of 55 or less** are **slow-release carbohydrates** and are the best choices for most people. This is particularly true for inactive people, the overweight, sportsmen and women before exercise, as well as diabetics, hypoglycaemics, people suffering from hyperinsulinaemia, insulin resistance, candidiasis, polycystic ovarian syndrome (PCOS), ME, FMS, inflammatory disease such as arthritis, high triglycerides and AD(H)D (Attention Deficit [Hyperactivity] Disorder). Slow-release carbohydrates do not result in a sudden, high rise in blood glucose levels, and for this reason they keep blood glucose levels steady for several hours. **They are called low GI foods.** Low GI foods are more satisfying and do not cause the release of as much insulin as high GI foods do. Low GI foods, therefore, also prevent the huge drop in blood glucose levels which usually occurs after the initial rapid rise in blood glucose levels after eating high GI foods. High GI foods elicit a huge insulin response, the body's way of coping with the sudden, sharp rise in blood glucose levels. Often the insulin response is too much, and blood glucose levels fall rapidly to below the starting point, a condition known as hypoglycaemia. This swing from very high to very low blood glucose levels, due to hyperinsulinaemia, is now believed to be a contributing factor to most of the so-called lifestyle diseases. These diseases are actually caused by high insulin levels in the blood, and could be prevented, to a large extent, if the general public were to consume lower fat, lower GI foods most of the time and reserve higher GI foods for during and/or after exercise, depending on the duration and intensity of exercise. Researchers regard all foods with a GI of 62 or below as 'safe', even though the theoretical cut-off point for a low GI food is 55.

Intermediate and high GI foods, on the other hand, are very useful for sportsmen and women, during and after taking part in sport. **Intermediate GI foods** are those with a **GI ranging from 56 to 69, and release glucose moderately fast into the bloodstream.**

They are the best choice in the following cases:
- in healthy persons, after low intensity exercise of short duration, e.g. a brisk, 30-minute walk
- the morning after an evening of prolonged and vigorous exercise
- in diabetics, directly after moderate activity, such as 1 hour's training in a gym and during and immediately after exercise lasting longer then 1–1½ hours.

Foods with a GI of 70+ are **fast-release carbohydrates** and are called **high GI foods.** High GI foods are excellent for the prevention of fatigue and hypoglycaemia in regular sportsmen within 30–60 minutes of completing moderate to high-intensity exercise lasting at least 1 hour, and during and within 30–60 minutes of completing exercise lasting more than 1–1½ hours. High GI foods should, however, be avoided by diabetics under normal circumstances, but could perhaps be consumed during and after strenuous exercise, lasting 90 minutes or more, after

careful experimentation. Small quantities of high GI foods are also useful during a low blood glucose 'attack' (the so-called hypo), but it is better to prevent low blood glucose levels than to treat it.

Any person wishing to sustain energy during exercise should not consume high GI foods before exercise or when they are inactive, but should rather have low GI foods. (Please see page 19 for more detailed information on sports nutrition).

Healthy eating

In South Africa we now have Food-Based Dietary Guidelines which are really easy to understand and implement on a daily basis (see below). By simply applying the first guideline – eating a variety of foods at every meal – you ensure a wide variety of nutrients, which in turn optimises nutrition. Applying all of them would optimise your nutritional intake, and the recipes in this book do just that.

South African Dietary Guidelines

1   Enjoy a variety of foods.
2   Be active.
3   Make lower GI starchy foods the basis of most meals.
4   Eat plenty of vegetables and fruits every day.
5   Eat cooked dried beans, peas, lentils and soya regularly.
6   Lower fat chicken, fish, meat, milk, yoghurt, cheese or eggs could be eaten daily.
7   Eat fats (especially saturated fats) sparingly.
8   Use salt sparingly, and limit salty foods.
9   Drink lots of clean, safe water.
10 If you drink alcohol, drink sensibly, i.e. not more than 1–2 drinks per day.
11 Eat and drink foods containing sugar sparingly, and not between meals.

Breakfast is the most important meal of the day and 'sets the stage', in a manner of speaking, for the rest of the day. This is particularly true for diabetic persons. A well-balanced lower GI, lower fat breakfast has a stabilising effect on blood glucose levels, so that by the time lunch time comes around, you are only just hungry again and have not had a blood glucose surge or slump all morning.

In other words, the body has been able to operate with optimum fuel levels all morning. A high GI and/or high fat breakfast can result in shakiness, fatigue and irritability all day long, unless a substantial amount of exercise was done before breakfast and the high GI breakfast was consumed within 30–60 minutes of completing the exercise. This is due to the excess insulin released in response to the surge in blood glucose from the high GI food, which does not happen after exercise, due to the action of the enzyme, glycogen resynthetase, which is very active after exercise and which is responsible for replacing the glycogen lost from the muscles and liver during exercise.

Breakfast

We would like, therefore, to recommend that those who don't exercise before breakfast eat a hearty lower fat, lower GI breakfast to keep blood glucose levels stable for the rest of the morning. Breakfast should contain lower GI carbohydrate foods e.g. a lower GI muffin, or cereal or porridge (see GI list on page 22), some protein, e.g. lower fat cheese, and a little fat (already in the muffin and cheese). Fruit can either be added to the breakfast or eaten as a mid-morning snack. See pages 24–28 for breakfast ideas.

Lunch / Light meals

The modern trend is not to eat lunch. This results in very low blood glucose levels before supper time, and the result is often a raid on the fridge. We'd like to emphasise, therefore, the importance of eating a lower fat, lower GI lunch, consisting mainly of lower GI starch, e.g. seed loaf (see GI list on page 22 for more lower GI options), as well as salad. Add to this a little lower fat protein or dairy, e.g. lean meat/fish/chicken/cheese/eggs/legumes, and a minimum of fat, e.g. spread avocado on your bread instead of margarine. End off the meal with low GI fruit, or keep the fruit for a snack later on. For lunch-time suggestions see the sections on light meals (pages 38–46), salads (pages 34–36) and soups (pages 30–32).

Supper or dinner / Main meals

The bulk of the evening meal should, once again, be lower GI carbohydrates, in the form of vegetables and starch. Approximately half of your plate should be filled with vegetables, one-quarter with low GI starch (see GI list on page 22) and only one-quarter with lower fat protein (lean meat, fish or chicken; or beans, peas, lentils or texturised vegetable protein). Vegetarians can eat low-fat milk, yoghurt, cheese, legumes or nuts as protein, but should remember that nuts are 50% fat and their intake should therefore be limited, even though they contain mainly healthier fat. (See main meals [pages 48–84] and light meals [pages 35–46]).

Eating high GI carbohydrates for supper, after a day of non-activity, could result in reactive low blood glucose levels a few hours later or during the night. Diabetic persons who eat high GI starches for supper, will invariably have elevated blood glucose levels above 10 mmol/l about 1 hour after supper, and elevated fasting blood glucose levels the next morning, i.e. over 7 mmol/l, both of which are undesirable.

Eating protein with higher GI carbohydrates will reduce the effect of the carbohydrates on blood glucose levels, but not as effectively as when higher GI carbohydrates are eaten together with proteins that contain carbohydrates and have an overall low GI, e.g. low-fat milk, yoghurt and legumes. See the discussion on the Glycaemic load (GL) on page 10. Eating large portions of protein and fat, such as fatty red meat, can also result in high blood glucose levels the next morning, especially in those with diabetes.

Fibre

Most South Africans do not even come close to the recommended 30–40 g fibre per day. Low fibre intakes have been linked to high cholesterol levels, high blood pressure, diabetes (since most high-fibre foods – although not all of them – are also low GI and in addition, fibre also improves insulin sensitivity), spastic colon and cancer, especially colon and breast cancer.

Fibre is the indigestible part of plant foods, and is therefore not found in animal protein or fats. It moves almost untouched through the alimentary canal until it reaches the colon, adding bulk and softness to the stool for easy evacuation. There are two types of fibre: water-soluble fibre found in oats, oat bran, barley, legumes, pasta, mealies, deciduous and citrus fruits and some vegetables, and insoluble fibre, found in digestive bran, brown and whole-wheat bread, whole-wheat (sold as Weet-Rice or pearled wheat), brown rice, etc. Both play a vital role in gut health, and should be consumed every day.

Foods that contain mainly soluble fibre usually have a low GI. If eaten regularly instead of high fat, high GI foods, they can protect against Type 2 Diabetes, since these foods do not over-stimulate insulin secretion. Constant over-stimulation of insulin secretion by eating high fat, high GI, low-fibre foods may lead to the depletion of the beta cells of the pancreas, which are responsible for producing insulin and the onset of Type 2 Diabetes. Soluble fibre also binds cholesterol, and is therefore effective in lowering cholesterol levels.

Although we include some low-fibre foods in the GI list on pages 22–23, so that you can know which foods are low, intermediate and high GI, we want to encourage you rather to choose a higher fibre product that is also lower in fat and GI, instead of the refined counterpart.

The sweet truth about sugar

When one hears the word 'sugar', one automatically thinks of table sugar, the sweetness we add to tea and coffee. There is much more to sugar than that, however. Chemically, sugar is known as sucrose, but technically there are many different types of sugar. For example, the sugar in fruit can be fructose, sucrose, glucose, or a combination of any of these; the sugar in milk is lactose, and so on. A sugar-free food may, in fact, not be sugar free at all – merely free of sucrose, and it is not necessarily low GI or lower in kilojoules. New SA legislation may not allow for a food to be called 'sugar free' if it contains any of the types of sugars listed below unless the GI has been tested.

A. SUGARS: MONO- AND DISACCHARIDES: These consist of either 1 or 2 molecules of different sugars and have varying effects on blood glucose levels or the Glycaemic Index (GI) of the food containing them. Some (low GI) are absorbed more slowly and steadily than others, which can be absorbed really rapidly (high GI).

The following 'sugars' individually have a low GI, but contain just as many kilojoules (kJ) as table sugar: fructose,

Krystar 300 (fructose), Fructofin C (fructose – GMO free), Dolcresun Q0 & Q2 (a syrup that's very high in fructose) and lactose (milk sugar).

The following 'sugars' have an intermediate GI and contain as many kilojoules as the above: sucrose (table sugar) and invert sugar.

The following 'sugars' are high GI and contain as many kilojoules as table sugar: glucose, dextrose, maltose and maltotriose.

B. Sugar alcohols/Polyols (1–2 molecules): These also consist of 2 molecules of different sugars, but are, in addition, bound to an alcohol molecule. This makes them more difficult to digest, which means the sugar is released into the bloodstream more slowly, resulting in a low GI value. A certain percentage of these sugars is not digested at all, and thus they contain less kilojoules than regular sugars. They can, however, cause gastric discomfort (flatulence, cramping and/or diarrhoea), if taken in excess.

Examples of sugar alcohols are: lactitol, xylitol, isomalt, maltitol, sorbitol and mannitol.

C. Oligosaccharides (3–9 molecules): These consist of more than 2 molecules of different sugars and can be either low GI or high GI.

Indigestible oligosaccharides (low GI) are not digested at all, and the body deals with them as it would deal with fibre. All of them are, therefore, low GI, and most are also kilojoule free, except for Sugalite, which contains about ⅓ of the kilojoules of table sugar. These sugars ferment in the colon and form short-chain fatty acids. This has certain health benefits, such as a reduction in fasting blood glucose, but they can also cause gastric discomfort if taken in excess (flatulence, cramping and/or diarrhoea). Examples of oligosaccharides include Frutafit HD, IQ and TEX, Inulin (FOS or fructo-oligosaccharides), polydextrose, Litesse Ultra (ultra-refined polydextrose), Litesse II (refined polydextrose), pyrodextrins, galacto-olgisaccharides, raffinose, stachyose and Sugalite.

Some malto-oligosaccharides (high GI), such as maltodextrin, can be digested by our bodies, but contain as many kilojoules as table sugar, and have a very high GI value, i.e. over 100!

D. Polysaccharides (>10 molecules): These contain as many kilojoules as table sugar, and most of them are high GI. Examples of these are: dextrins – which are intermediate products in the hydrolysis of starch, and consist of shorter chains of glucose units, and glucose polymers or corn syrup solids, which are partially or fully hydrolysed cornstarch.

E. Non-nutritive or artificial sweeteners: These are the only sweeteners that are free of energy or kilojoules. Do not eat them too freely though, as we are not sure of their long-term effects on the human body. Examples: saccharine, cyclamates,

acesulfame K, aspartame and sucralose.

Now you know how to distinguish between the effects of different 'sugars' on blood glucose levels, as well as their kilojoule value. If any of the high GI 'sugars' listed above are one of the first 3 ingredients in a product, beware! The GI might just be high.

Conditions that benefit from the lower GI, lower fat way of eating

Diabetes mellitus

Diabetes is on the increase, at a rate of 11% a year, and there is talk of an epidemic of diabetes. This is due in part to the high GI, high fat diet the general public consumes, as well as an increasingly sedentary lifestyle, stress and smoking.

There are 2 types of diabetes: Type 1 diabetes (10% of diabetics) and Type 2 diabetes (90% of diabetics). In Type I diabetes, the beta cells of the pancreas are unable to produce insulin and the onset is usually sudden. A pre-existing genetic component is usually present, as well as a precipitating factor, e.g. a viral infection or, in some cases, certain proteins which can spark off an immune response. Often, it is the trigger that is the proverbial last straw for becoming diabetic, e.g. an infection, stress or trauma. These do not, however, *cause* diabetes.

The classic symptoms, especially of Type 1 diabetes, include chronic thirst, chronic urination, chronic hunger and excessive weight loss in spite of consuming large quantities of food and drink. Type I diabetics need to inject insulin every day.

Type 2 diabetes is less easy to diagnose and the onset is usually slow. Thirty percent of Type 2 diabetics already have complications at the time of diagnosis. Usually these people are overweight, have insulin resistance and already have high cholesterol and/or high triglyceride levels, as well as high blood pressure by the time diabetes is diagnosed. They often have no, or vague, symptoms, e.g. chronic infections, chronic fatigue, pain, cramps or a burning sensation in the legs and feet, shortness of breath, etc. Some of these people have a relative insulin deficiency and can be treated with diet and exercise alone, or diet, exercise and tablets. Others have an absolute insulin shortage and need to be treated with diet, exercise and insulin therapy. Early diagnosis is important, so have your blood glucose, blood lipids and blood pressure checked regularly irrespective of symptoms. The earlier diabetes is diagnosed and treated, the smaller the chances are of serious complications.

Modern treatment of diabetes

As with all new research, the Glycaemic Index (GI) has not been universally welcomed with open arms. It has its critics, most of whom cling to past assumptions. Unfortunately, they prefer to believe what they think should happen to a person's blood glucose in response to eating certain foods, rather than having to face what actually happens to blood glucose when carbohydrate-rich foods are eaten. The GI, remember, is a physiological measure of the body's response to a particular carbohydrate-rich food.

Research conducted over the past 20 years in Canada, Australia, the United Kingdom, Italy, France, Denmark, the East and Far East, as well as South Africa, shows convincingly that many foods that were regarded as 'safe' on the traditional sugar-free diet, actually raise diabetic persons' blood glucose levels higher than some ordinary foods that may contain a little sugar. Some of the foods previously regarded as 'safe' elicit very high blood glucose level increases and should rather be avoided. Many other foods that contain sugar, which diabetic persons have had to avoid in the past, cause no major fluctuations in blood glucose levels. It does not, therefore, make sense to ban these foods for those with diabetes. If you consult the GI list (page 22), you will notice that South African brown bread has a high GI value, whereas sweetened fruit yoghurt has a low GI value. This means that one or two slices of brown bread, eaten as dry toast, for example, will result in a much greater blood glucose level rise than eating a small tub of sweetened fruit yoghurt.

The new lower fat, lower GI diet is much more effective in lowering and controlling blood glucose levels, because it is based on what happens to real people (diabetics and non-diabetics) when they eat real food, in real life. Umpteen dieticians across the world have countless examples of how diabetics' insulin and oral medication can be decreased – or even discontinued in some cases – when the lower GI, lower fat diet is followed. Many of these people had been on a sugar-free diet (and sometimes even low fat as well) for many years and still could not get their blood glucose readings under 10 mmol/l. As soon as they go on the lower fat, lower GI diet, their readings are less than 10 mmol/l for the first time in years – not by avoiding sugar, but by avoiding high fat, high GI foods.

A high-fat diet also results in the insulin working less effectively, which, in turn, can lead to a relative or absolute shortage of insulin, hyperinsulinaemia and insulin resistance. This predisposes a person to all the lifestyle diseases (diabetes, heart disease, hypertension and overweight). The lower fat, lower GI diet is much more 'user friendly' than the standard diabetic diet, because sugar is no longer completely forbidden. Portion control is no longer so important when eating slow-release (lower GI), lower fat foods, as the increased satiety automatically controls how much one eats. If you are overweight, however, you will still have to watch portion sizes. This is the reason we give the amount of starch, protein, fat, etc. for every recipe: so that those who want or need to watch their weight can to do so by sticking to the recommended portion quantities given to them by a dietician. In addition, keeping to the number of servings recommended per dish at the top of every recipe, will also help with weight management. Larger portion sizes are, however, also given for those whose weight is normal or who need to carbo-load or gain weight.

Please note that all the recipes in this book are suitable for all diabetics. Every meal consumed by a diabetic should contain at least one low GI food (slow-release carbohydrates). If most of the foods in a meal are low GI, then intermediate (and even small quantities of high) GI foods can be added to the same meal. We applied this principle in many of the recipes in this book, and have mentioned this in the Dietician's notes. For maximum reduction in blood glucose levels – especially if you have a fasting blood glucose value that is higher than 8 mmol/l and a random blood glucose that is higher than 10 mmol/l – it is important to consume mainly low GI foods at every meal.

Hypoglycaemia (low blood sugar)

Hypoglycaemia is a condition in which blood glucose levels fall below normal levels (hypo = under and glycaemia = blood sugar/glucose). Many people suffer from hypoglycaemia, not surprisingly since most of the foods that are freely available and consumed by the general public are high in fat and have a high GI value. The most common form of hypoglycaemia occurs after a meal or snack is eaten. This is called reactive hypoglycaemia. High GI foods (except when eaten during or after exercise), result in a sharp increase in blood glucose levels within a short period of time, i.e. 15–30 minutes after eating. The human body then tries to rectify the situation by releasing insulin to counteract the threat of sustained high blood glucose levels. Insulin removes the glucose from the bloodstream, often too enthusiastically, resulting in a rapid fall in blood glucose levels. The end result is the typical stress-like symptoms of low blood sugar levels, i.e. tremors, heart palpitations, sweating, anxiety, irritability, sleepiness, weakness and shakiness, as well as the very common feeling of chronic fatigue. Hypoglycaemia can also affect mental function and lead to restlessness, irritability, poor concentration, visual disturbance, lethargy and drowsiness. These symptoms are clearly noticeable in non-diabetics during GI research undertaken by scientists, especially if high GI foods are eaten.

The logical treatment for hypoglycaemia is to control the influx of glucose into the bloodstream. Consuming mainly slow-release carbohydrates (low GI) at meals and as snacks, one is able to ensure a slow, but steady stream of glucose being released into the bloodstream that will not trigger the release of huge surges of insulin. If, on top of eating high GI foods, one consumes a lot of fat, especially saturated fat (which causes the body's insulin to work less effectively), it is only a question of time before impaired glucose tolerance (the forerunner of Type 2 diabetes) develops. The reason for this is that the body's insulin is depleted by continually trying to correct the surges of glucose released into the blood when fast-release carbohydrates (high GI) are eaten, and the insulin that's left cannot work properly due to the high-fat diet. This can lead to hyperinsulinaemia (too much insulin in the blood, in response to the high blood glucose levels) and insulin resistance. Insulin resistance causes the body's cells to shut down (since they do not like to be drowned in insulin) and 'forget' that they are supposed to transfer the glucose from the bloodstream to the body cells, in response to insulin. The results are high insulin, as well as high blood glucose levels. Other factors that can contribute to insulin resistance are genetic factors, inactivity, obesity and ageing. Hyperinsulinaemia, in turn, can lead to diabetes, hyperlipidaemia, hypertension and heart disease, as well as resistant overweight or obesity. This whole vicious cycle needs to be broken before the body will start functioning properly again.

Follow these simple guidelines to prevent hypoglycaemia and all its nasty consequences:
• Eat regular meals and snacks, preferably every 3 hours.
• Include slow-release carbohydrates (low GI) at every meal or snack to keep blood glucose levels steady.

Avoid eating fast-release carbohydrates (high GI) on their own, unless taken after exercise or during and after prolonged exercise. Preferably avoid them altogether (see GI list on page 22), but if you have to eat a high GI carbohydrate, always combine it with low GI carbohydrates or at least with some protein. Eating high and low GI foods together yields an overall intermediate GI, as explained previously.

For lots of tips on food combining, see *The South African Glycaemic Index Guide*, GIFSA, 2002.

Sport-induced hypoglycaemia

Hypoglycaemia or 'low blood sugar' occurring during or after sport, can happen when the sportsman or woman does not eat slow-release carbohydrate foods (low GI) before exercise and either eats nothing during and/or after exercise, or eats slow-release foods (low GI) during and/or after exercise, or eats too long after exercise. To prevent this, low GI carbohydrates (slow release) should be eaten 1–2 hours before exercise in order to stabilise blood glucose and insulin levels during exercise. Higher GI beverages or food (fast release) should be consumed within the first 30–60 minutes after exercise lasting 1–1½ hours, and during and after exercise lasting longer than 1–1½ hours. Doing this keeps blood glucose levels steady and replenishes glycogen used by the muscles.

Coronary heart disease (CHD)

In westernised South Africans, 40% of deaths in the economically active age group (25–64 years), result from chronic lifestyle diseases, such as cancer, hypertension (high blood pressure), diabetes, strokes and coronary heart disease or CHD. Of all these, CHD causes the greatest number of deaths. In fact, CHD is the number-one killer in South Africa, and many other countries worldwide, today. The development of CHD is a slow process and starts with a fatty deposit build-up on the inner walls of the arteries of the heart and brain. This may lead to narrowing and hardening of the arteries (arteriosclerosis) that supply the heart and the brain with oxygen. When the blood can no longer get through, the person suffers a heart attack or stroke. Often, a part of the heart muscle dies, or a section of the body is paralysed (stroke), if the patient is lucky enough to survive. The frightening thing is that, as excess cholesterol slowly constricts and clogs your arteries, you won't necessarily suffer any pain or discomfort, except maybe fatigue and shortness of breath. Some people experience chest pain (angina), but for many, the first warning sign could be a heart attack or stroke.

Risk factors

A number of factors contribute to an increased risk of CHD, including high blood cholesterol levels, high blood pressure, being overweight, diabetes, smoking, stress, a lack of exercise, a family history of CHD, to name some of them. An increasing number of people have also been found to suffer from high levels of blood triglycerides (another type of fat in the blood that predisposes one to diabetes). To lower such higher triglyceride levels, a lower fat, low Glycaemic load diet is recommended. High levels of blood cholesterol and triglycerides, high blood pressure, diabetes, being overweight, gout and cancer are all influenced by the quantity of fat (especially saturated fat and 'processed' fat) in our diet. Higher saturated fat intakes result in more LDL cholesterol, which is the dangerous cholesterol. Oxidised LDL cholesterol is laid down in the arteries most easily and that is why it is important to prevent oxidation of LDL cholesterol by eating lots of fresh fruit and vegetables. Saturated fat also causes the body to retain dietary cholesterol, which makes saturated fat the number-one culprit in raising blood cholesterol levels, not dietary cholesterol, as was previously thought. It can also reduce levels of the good HDL cholesterol, which is another reason saturated fat (animal fats) should be restricted. Fat, especially saturated fat, is also believed to be the main dietary promoter of cancer, as well as the main cause of extra body fat or obesity. Most of the foods South Africans love to eat are high in saturated fats and trans-fatty acids, another 'bad' fat. To name but a few: fatty meat such as lamb and mutton chops, dried sausage, fatty biltong, toasted sandwiches, pies and other confectionery such as cakes, tarts, biscuits, rusks and croissants, full-cream ice cream, chocolate, rich sauces, desserts and all deep-fried foods. Too much sodium, together with a high fat, high GI diet, too much alcohol, and being overweight and inactive can aggravate high blood pressure.

Treatment

It is, however, possible to eat most of these foods, provided they are the lower fat, lower GI and lower sodium version. This book is full of delicious, normal recipes that are low in total fat, saturated fat, trans-fatty acids, GI, GL and sodium, and will not cause fatty deposit build-up on the inner walls of arteries.

We decided to recommend the use of canola or olive oil (which are both high in mono-unsaturated fats) in the recipes, as research has shown that large quantities of omega-6 polyunsaturated fatty acids (PUFAs), especially those of plant origin – e.g. polyunsaturated soft (tub) margarine, sunflower oil, cottonseed oil, sunflower seeds, walnuts, etc. – can give rise to nasty reactive chemicals called free radicals, which are implicated in heart disease, cancer and ageing, and can lessen the more beneficial HDL cholesterol. Polyunsaturated fats (omega 3s) which occur in fatty fish, e.g. pilchards, trout, tuna (packed in water or brine), sardines and salmon (without the oil), mackerel (in water), etc. seem to be much healthier, since they lower fibrinogen levels in the blood, which slows down blood clotting, and also helps to increase the good HDL cholesterol. We recommend that fatty fish be eaten once or twice a week.

Monounsaturated fats, which are found in olive oil, canola oil, macadamia oil, olives, avocados, peanut butter and raw un-salted nuts (except brazil nuts) reduce bad cholesterol and raise good HDL cholesterol levels. HDL cholesterol is responsible for the removal of the 'bad' fats from the arteries, by transporting them to the liver to be excreted. HDL cholesterol levels may be raised by exercise, a low GI diet, wise consumption of red wine (1–2 wine glasses per day) and using mainly mono-unsaturated and omega-3 polyunsaturated fats as sources of fat.

Fibre, especially soluble fibre (which happens to be in many low GI foods, such as legumes, barley and oat bran), also plays an important role in decreasing the risk of CHD. Soluble fibre binds cholesterol in the alimentary canal, thereby reducing serum cholesterol, especially the bad LDL cholesterol. For this reason we have included many recipes with one or other legume or lower GI oats/oat bran as an ingredient. The plant sterols in legumes are very effective at decreasing the risk of heart disease and oat products are the richest sources of solu-ble fibre. If you want to reduce the risk of CHD, you will have to exercise more, stop smoking, decrease your intake of salt, lose weight or avoid becoming overweight, and eat a lower fat, lower GI diet.

Attention Deficit Hyperactivity Disorder (ADHD) or Attention Deficit Disorder (ADD)

For years it was believed that ADHD and ADD were caused, or at least aggravated, by the consumption of sugar. Sugar was believed to cause hypoglycaemia, and it was recently found that hyperactivity and/or ADHD and hypoglycaemia are interrelated. Now that we know that it is high Glycaemic Index (GI) foods that cause hypoglycaemia, we recommend that children who suffer from ADHD or ADD should avoid high GI foods (such as refined bread, most refined cereals, cold drinks, energy drinks and sweets that are high in glucose), rather than just avoiding foods that are high in sugar.

Why ADHD, ADD and hypoglycaemia are interrelated

Many children with ADHD or ADD crave high GI carbohydrates. All high GI foods cause a rapid rise in blood glucose levels, which results in the pancreas pouring out insulin in an attempt to bring the blood glucose down to a normal level. In many people, and some children who suffer from ADHD or ADD, the body pours out too much insulin, resulting in too much glucose being drawn out of the blood, and the blood sugar level falling below normal.

The end result is a hypoglycaemic attack with the accompany-ing irritability, poor sleeping habits and lack of concentration. (See the section on hypoglycaemia, page 15, for other symp-toms that are usually caused by eating high GI foods.) When high GI foods are eaten for breakfast, a hypo-glycaemic attack may occur 1–1½ hours later – before first break at school, and at a time when the brain should still be receiving a steady supply of energy from the food eaten 2–3 hours earlier, as is the case with low GI foods. If high GI foods are eaten at break (which often happens, since the child feels the need to compensate for the tired feeling by eating, usually another high GI food), the same scenario can repeat itself later in the morning. This, we think, is the reason these children struggle to concentrate. The brain's fuel is constantly undergoing huge swings and this is not conducive to thinking or behaving in a normal manner.

Evidence is starting to emerge that an adverse food reaction may also cause a significant drop in blood glucose levels. The endocrine (glandular) system overreacts and this may cause a sudden rise – and later a drop – in blood glucose levels. It is hypothesised that, by constantly eating certain foods, the enzymes needed to digest and metabolise the food are over-extended, to the point where an allergy to that particular food may develop. When an allergic reaction develops, a chemi-cal called histamine can be produced. Histamine causes the adrenal glands to excrete adrenalin, which stimulates the liver to convert stored sugar (glycogen) into blood glucose. This sudden rise in blood sugar levels can also cause the pancreas to pour out insulin. The end result is a hypoglycaemic attack. If a child is allergic to a specific food, it can also cause hypoglycaemia and swings in blood glucose levels and moods. The fact that allergy to a specific foodstuff affects blood glucose levels has been confirmed by GI tests, and we have also observed this in some of our patients.

Caffeine can also cause hyperactivity initially, and hypo-glycaemia with the resultant symptoms later. This is due to the fact that caffeine also stimulates the adrenal glands to excrete adrenalin, which stimulates the liver to pour glucose into the bloodstream. This sudden rise in blood sugar levels can once again cause the pancreas to pour out insulin. The end result is a hypoglycaemic attack.

Treatment

In light of the above, we recommend that all high GI foods, caffeine and any food to which a child with ADHD or ADD is allergic, should be avoided, as all these foods may induce hy-poglycaemia. If low GI foods are eaten most of the time, but especially for breakfast (since breakfast sets the tone for the rest of the day), the brain receives a steady supply of energy from the food. This is because low GI foods result neither in a sudden, nor a substantial rise in blood glucose levels, and consequently no sudden drop in blood glucose levels, due to the over-secretion of insulin. Low GI foods keep blood glucose levels even enabling the child to concentrate better. Examples of low GI breakfast foods include: lower GI oats, whole-wheat ProNutro, high-fibre cereal, deciduous fruits and fruit yoghurt, to name but a few. (See the GI list [page 22] and the breakfast section [pages 24–28]) for more ideas.

It is also advisable to keep these children away from flavourants, preservatives, and especially colourants, since the latter was found to inhibit the brain's uptake of a very important neurotransmitter, vital for the transmission of messages. Foods and medicines containing salicylate should also preferably be avoided, since they are chemically related to the former 3 additives and can interfere with the transmission of messages in the brain. Children who suffer from ADHD or ADD also benefit greatly from additional essential fatty acids (especially omega-3 fatty acids, which enhance the transfer of messages in the brain), as well as certain vitamins and minerals. For more information, consult a dietician who specialises in the treatment of ADHD. See GIFSA's website at www.gifoundation.com for a complete list of dieticians who use the GI in their treatment of patients.

The only exception to the low GI rule is during, and especially after, exercise, but more about that in the section on sports nutrition (page 19).

Please note that all the recipes in this book are suitable for children with ADHD and ADD, provided that the child does not suffer from an allergy to one of the ingredients, and is not salicylate sensitive.

Weight management

For a complete guide to effective weight management see our book, *Eat Smart and Stay Slim: The GI Diet.*

Follow a lower fat diet

For some unknown reason, carbohydrates (CHO) have, for the last 20–30 years, been labelled fattening. Although research undertaken in the last 10 years has disproved this over and again, carbohydrates are still struggling to get rid of the 'fattening' label. Carbohydrate has actually been found to stimulate its own metabolism, which means that if you eat more, your body will merely burn more.

This is, however, not the case with fat. Dietary fat has been found simply to slip into body fat unchanged, proving that it does not stimulate its own metabolism. If one eats a lot of a certain type of fat (such as that in chocolate), the fat in one's body will look exactly like chocolate fat. If, on the other hand, one eats a lot of cheese, the fat in one's body will look exactly like the fat in cheese.

In a British study, scientists isolated a number of people in a room for a week, allowing them to eat low-fat or fat-free carbohydrates to their hearts' content. After a week, these people had only gained a maximum of 1.5 kg. When these same people were isolated and allowed to eat high-fat foods to their hearts' desire, some of them picked up as much as 7 kg! This shows

clearly that in order to lose weight (or rather fat), one needs to cut down on one's intake of visible and hidden fats.

All the recipes in this book are much lower in fat than ordinary recipes and we also show you, in the choice of ingredients and preparation methods, how to decrease the fat content of all meals and snacks. Do not, however, avoid fat altogether. One needs a small quantity of 'good' fats in the diet so that you will ingest all the essential fatty acids – needed for their favourable effect on blood lipids and the skin, as well as to prevent cravings due to overly strict dieting.

Eat regular, small meals

Regular, smaller, snack-type meals are recommended to lose weight and stay slim. Do not, however end up eating all the time! Increased insulin secretion is stimulated when large meals are eaten, and insulin plays a role in how we store fat. Hyperinsulinaemia (too much insulin) is a major contributor to overweight, high body fat levels and the inability to lose weight. To facilitate weight loss and stay slim, it is therefore of the utmost importance that there should be no major increase in insulin secretion. It is also important not to cut food intake too drastically, as any major cut in food intake, especially to levels below 4 200 kJ per day, usually leads to a slowing down of the metabolism. Less is not always best!

Eat lower GI foods

Another important aspect of weight loss is keeping blood glucose levels as stable as possible, and the best way to do this is to implement the concept of the Glycaemic Index (GI). In a South African study (reported in *The GI Factor*, by Jenny Brand Miller et al.), it was found that people on a low GI slimming diet lost 2 kg more over a period of 12 weeks than their counterparts on a high GI diet. What was astounding was that both groups were given exactly the same quantity of fat, kilojoules, protein, carbohydrates and fibre. The success of the low GI slimming diet was attributed to the fact that a low GI diet does not cause a major insulin response, resulting in lower insulin levels and more stable blood glucose levels. This, in turn, assists the body in losing body fat, which is prevented by high insulin levels. Whereas this might be true of a high carbohydrate, high GI diet this is not the case with a high carbohydrate, low GI diet. By avoiding high GI carbohydrates, except during and/or after exercise, and following the prudent diet (50–55% CHO, 30–35% fat and 12–20% protein), but eating mainly low GI carbohydrates, you will optimise body fat loss. Low GI carbohydrates also keep you feeling satisfied for longer, and prevent 'sweet cravings', unlike a high protein diet.

Exercise regularly

Regular exercise is an essential part of good health, and especially for successful weight management. It is, in fact, so important that the *SA Dietary Guidelines* (see page 12) places exercise second on the list, even though it is not, strictly speaking, a dietary guideline! Exercise increases lean body mass, which in turn increases the metabolism. Trying to slim without exercising regularly can lead to muscle loss, because the body finds it easier to turn muscle into energy than to burn body fat for energy, leading to a slowing down of the metabolism. This is especially true if the food intake is cut drastically. So, to lose fat most effectively, don't do anything drastic! Forget about dieting and just eat ordinary lower fat, lower GI meals (except after exercise) and exercise daily. Your eating plan for weight management must be one you can follow for the rest of your life. But watch the size of your portions; you won't lose weight if you eat too much, even if you are eating the right foods. To help you, we have included portion sizes with each recipe. And be patient: it takes time to burn fat!

Find out why you eat

If you eat for emotional, physical or circumstancial reasons, instead of in response to your body's needs (i.e. true hunger), you will have to tackle these reasons, otherwise you will never get slim and maintain your weight. (See *Eat Smart and Stay Slim: The GI diet*, to find out whether you are a compulsive eater.)

Sports nutrition

The only exception to the low GI guideline, is during and/or after exercise. Generally speaking, to sustain energy, we should all eat low GI carbohydrate foods most of the time. Sportsmen and women, however, should eat low GI carbohydrates (1 g carbohydrate per 1 kg body weight) 1–2 hours before exercise, and then only resume low GI eating a couple of hours after completing the exercise, depending on its duration and intensity.

It is best to consume high GI carbohydrate foods and drinks during, immediately after, and for a few hours after exercise, once again depending on the duration and intensity. Intermediate GI foods during and/or after exercise are recommended for the diabetic sportsman or woman, and those who have a blood sugar (glucose) sensitivity.

Pre-sport or event

Consume 1 g low GI carbohydrate per 1 kg body weight, 1–2 hours before exercise. Low GI foods and drinks release glucose slowly and steadily, so they maintain a healthy 'petrol' level during the activity or sporting event.

During the event

Competitions or training sessions that last for more than 60–90 minutes require high GI foods and drinks (intermediate for diabetics and those with sensitive blood sugar) at a rate of 30–60 g CHO per hour, depending on body weight. If the duration of the exercise is less than 60–90 minutes, the low GI food or drink that was taken beforehand should be sufficient to sustain blood glucose at a healthy level, and only water need be consumed, at a rate of 250–500 ml (1–2 c) per hour.

Post-sport/event

It is crucial to consume at least 1 g of high GI (intermediate for diabetics) carbohydrate per 1 kg body weight within the first 30–60 minutes of completing exercise. Thereafter, 1 g lower GI carbohydrate per 1 kg body weight should be consumed every 2 hours after exercise. The reason for this is that the exercised muscles continue to absorb glucose from the bloodstream, and this happens at the fastest rate during the first 30–60 minutes after exercise. The replenishment of glycogen into the fatigued muscle is faster if higher GI foods are taken as soon as possible after exercise ends, due to the action of the enzyme glycogen resynthetase. Doing this can prevent severe hypoglycaemia, and one should also be ensured of sustained energy levels and replenished glycogen levels in the muscles and liver. Consuming some protein with the carbohydrate directly after exercise, will ensure full body muscle recovery.

For very active people, i.e. those who train 2–3 hours every morning, or an hour every morning and an hour every evening, it may mean having to eat intermediate to high GI foods most of the time. If, however, training is scaled down before an event, low GI carbohydrates should dominate all meals for the best carbo-loading effect. Carbo-loading can enhance performance in some people, but not in all. It's a good idea to try out any dietary changes long before the event to prevent any gastro-intestinal discomfort that may result from the higher carbohydrate intake. Basically, what this involves is eating a higher carbohydrate diet during the last 3 days before competing. For example, eating low GI cereals, bread (with jam), fruit and fruit juices for breakfast, and substituting pasta (macaroni, spaghetti, etc.) for some of your meat at suppertime, but still including lots of vegetables.

How sportsmen and women should use this book

The recipes in this book are all lower GI and suitable for daily consumption. Those suitable for carbo-loading before a sports event are clearly marked in the Dietician's notes provided with each recipe. Sportsmen and women who need high GI meals after their sports activity can substitute a high GI carbohydrate for a low GI carbohydrate in most of the recipes in this book; this will convert the meal into a low-fat, higher GI meal. For example, higher GI rice or high GI potatoes may be used instead of lower GI rice. Sportsmen should still eat low-fat meals, but high GI foods are required during, and for a few hours after, exercise, depending on its duration and intensity.

Vegetarians

Last, but not least, this recipe book is also suitable for vegetarians. All the recipes – except for a few main courses and light meals that contain meat, fish and chicken – are suitable, and many of these meals can be turned into vegetarian dishes simply by replacing the meat, fish or chicken with 1 or 2 cans of beans (1 can of cooked beans is equivalent to 250 ml [1 c] home-cooked dry beans). One entire section of the main courses contains recipes that do not call for meat, fish or chicken. These recipes teach the inexperienced vegetarian how to incorporate beans and legumes into meals in a tasty way, without the beans dominating the entire meal, and ensuring at the same time that the meals are nutritionally balanced. Many vegetarians are not sure how and what to eat. These recipes teach vegetarians how to make vegetarian meals that do not compromise good nutrition. Please note that a large percentage of the vegetarian dishes in most recipe books are high in fat. We had to limit the quantity of cheese and other sources of hidden fat in these recipes to ensure that every recipe complied with our lower fat recommendations.

Nutritional analysis of the recipes

You will notice that each recipe is accompanied by a box containing nutritional information. All the values have been rounded off to the nearest whole number. Each box contains the following information and reflects the amounts per serving:

GLYCAEMIC INDEX (GI) A calculated value. The value in real life will probably be lower, due to the interaction of the different nutrients with each other. The GI gives an indication of how quickly, and by how much, the food will affect blood glucose levels.

CARBOHYDRATE (g) This value gives the total carbohydrate (CHO) content per serving and includes the carbohydrate present in dairy, starch, vegetables and fruit.

PROTEIN (g) This represents the total amount of protein present per serving.

FAT (g) This value reflects the total fat content of the serving per person. Saturated fat and cholesterol values are not given, but they are kept low throughout.

FIBRE (g) The total quantity of fibre per serving, including soluble and insoluble fibre.

KILOJOULES (kJ) The total number of kilojoules (energy) per serving. To obtain calorie values, simply divide by 4.2.

GLYCAEMIC LOAD (GL) Reflects the 'oomph' or impact one portion of the dish will have on blood glucose levels, taking the amount of carbohydrate and GI into consideration. Recipes with a GL below 10 will have a minimal impact on blood glucose levels, even if the GI of the dish is intermediate or high. Recipes with higher GL values must be eaten in the recommended portion size to prevent a huge impact on blood glucose levels. The GL is a reflection of the GI, linked to the portion size of carbohydrate: the larger the portion, the higher the GL.

SODIUM Although we have not indicated the sodium content per serving, we did include it in our analysis, to make sure that all the recipes have a sodium content of less than 400 mg per serving; in fact, most of them are below 300 mg.

For each recipe, the portions of nutrients per serving are given. For example: ONE SERVING IS EQUIVALENT TO 1 STARCH + 1 PROTEIN.

(Consult a dietician if you want to know how many portions of starch, protein, fat, etc. you should consume per day. See www.gifoundation.com or www.diabetics.com)

The nutritional content of 1 portion for each food group is as follows:

- DAIRY The analysis for a low-fat Dairy portion applies: 523 kJ, 8 g protein, 5 g fat and 12 g carbohydrate.

  Where applicable, the analysis of a fat-free Dairy portion was used: 340 kJ, 8 g protein, 0 g fat and 12 g carbohydrate.
- PROTEIN The analysis for a medium-fat Protein portion applies: 328 kJ, 7 g protein and 5.5 g fat.
- LEAN PROTEIN The analysis for a virtually fat-free protein portion applies: 233 kJ, 7 g protein and 3 g fat.
- STARCH A Starch portion implies the following: 289 kJ, 15 g carbohydrate, 2 g protein and traces of fat.
- FAT A Fat portion implies the following: 190 kJ and 5 g fat.
- VEGETABLES The kilojoules and carbohydrates allocated to a limited Vegetable portion are: 153 kJ, 7 g carbohydrates and 2 g protein.

  When the kilojoule values allocated to the other food group portions in a recipe used up all the kilojoules, we did not count the kilojoules of the limited vegetables, even if the recipe contained some limited vegetable. Free vegetables contain less than 105 kJ per 100 g vegetables.
- FRUIT A Fruit portion implies the following: 255 kJ and 15 g carbohydrate.

MEASURES USED

In all the recipes in this book, the following measures (abbreviations in brackets) were used.

We used metric measuring spoons, measuring cups and measuring jugs.

¼ teaspoon (t) = 1 ml
½ teaspoon (t) = 2 ml
1 teaspoon (t) = 5 ml
2 teaspoons (t) = 10 ml
½ tablespoon (T) = 7 ml
1 tablespoon (T) = 15 ml
2 tablespoons (T) = 30 ml
¼ cup (c) = 65 ml
⅓ cup (c) = 85 ml
½ cup (c) = 125 ml
¾ cup (c) = 190 ml
1 cup (c) = 250 ml
2 cups (c) = 500 ml

GIFSA's lower fat, GI rated choice

The GIFSA lower fat GI rated choice is a range of logos that, if they appear on products or menus, indicate that these products are low(er) in fat, saturated fat, trans fatty acids and cholesterol; have a GI rating; allow a minimum of sodium; and also have fibre specifications. These ratings are offered in some restaurants and health shops in South Africa as a separate, lower GI, lower fat menu, and the GIFSA logo appears on some products in supermarkets. Listed below are the logos for the different ratings, with explanations.

Please refer to www.gifoundation.com for a glossary of relevant terms.

All the recipes in this book are lower in fat and have a lower GI value than regular recipes. The reason some recipes have an intermediate GI is due to the fact that they contain flour (and not necessarily due to their sugar content). All recipes, however, have a GI value of 62 or below, which the World Health Organisation (WHO) regards as 'safe' for all diabetics. The recipes in this book are endorsed by GIFSA, as indicated by the logo, which is their official endorsement mark.

The comprehensive *SA Glycaemic Index Guide* is available from the GI Foundation of SA (GIFSA) SA at www.gifoundation.com. It lists the GIs of most commonly eaten foods in South Africa, and also gives a comprehensive explanation of the Glycaemic Index, and how to practice food combining.

Wherever there is an asterisk (*) next to a product in a recipe, throughout the book, please refer to the Recommended Food/Product List (page 124) for a list of lower fat, lower GI products available in SA.

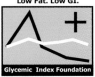**Frequent Foods** Low Fat. Low GI.	**GIFSA Green plus logo implies that the product** • can be eaten just about freely • is truly low in total fat (≤3 g fat/100 g food), low in saturated fat, trans-fatty acids and cholesterol • has a very low GI (≤40) • has a low sodium content and • has a high fibre content, where applicable
Often Foods Lower Fat. Low GI.	**GIFSA Green logo implies that the product** • can be eaten often, i.e. most of the time • is lower in total fat (≤10 g fat/100 g food), saturated fat, trans-fatty acids and cholesterol than its regular counterpart • has a low GI (≤55) • has a low sodium content and • has a moderate fibre content, where applicable
Special Treats Lower Fat. Intermediate GI.	**GIFSA Orange logo implies that the product** • should be kept for 'special treats' (people who have diabetes should preferably reserve it for after exercise lasting 1 hour, or during and after exercise lasting more than 1 hour) • may be slightly higher in total fat, saturated fat, trans-fatty acids and cholesterol, but still much lower in fat than its regular counterpart, i.e. it contains ≤15 g fat/100 g food • has an Intermediate GI, i.e. 56– 69GI (some of these products could have a low GI, but fall into this group due to a slightly higher fat content), and • has a moderately low sodium content
Best After Exercise Lower Fat. Higher GI.	**GIFSA Red logo implies that the product** • is best for regular sportsmen and women after exercise lasting 1 hour and during and after exercise lasting more than 1 hour • is low/moderate in fat, saturated fat, trans-fatty acids and cholesterol, but still much lower in fat than its regular counterpart i.e. it contains ≤15 g fat/100 g food • has a high GI value (70+) and • has a moderately low sodium content

The Glycaemic Index List of South African Lower Fat Foods

(The GI Value of glucose = 100)
Foods are listed in food groups, and in order of GI, starting with the lowest GI

Low GI (0–55)						
Dairy	**Cereals and porridges**	**Starches**	**Fruit**	**Vegetables**	**Sugars and snacks**	**Drinks**
MILK Low-fat or fat-free milk (plain and flavoured) Buttermilk, low-fat YOGHURT All low-fat and fat-free (plain and sweetened) CUSTARD Low-fat or fat-free (sweetened and unsweetened) ICE CREAM Low-fat (sweetened and unsweetened), e.g. Dialite ice cream	CEREALS ProNutro whole-wheat (Original and Apple Bake) ProNutro Original with low-fat milk Hi-Fibre Bran (Kellogg's) Fibre Plus Cereal (Bokomo) Shredded Bran Cereal (Pick 'n Pay) Fruitful All-Bran (Kellogg's) Bran Flakes (Bokomo) All Bran Flakes with skimmed milk (Kellogg's) Oat bran (raw) MUESLI Nature's Source muesli: Mixed Berries, Orange and Spices, Apple and Cinnamon Fine Form Muesli Morning Harvest Muesli (Bokomo) PORRIDGES Cooled mealie meal **Breads and Crackers** BREADS Bread containing lots of whole kernels, crushed wheat, oats and/or oat bran, e.g. seed loaves, pumper-nickel, Fine Form bread and Uncle Salie's seed loaf CRACKERS Bran crispbread Provita	PASTA All pasta made from durum wheat or durum wheat semolina Fine Form pastas LEGUMES Dried beans, peas and lentils, cooked or canned Baked beans RICE AND RICE SUBSTITUTES Pearled barley, whole and cracked Pearled wheat, whole (stampkoring or wheat rice) and cracked White (Tastic) Wild rice Brown rice (Old Mill Stream) CORN Whole corn (canned and frozen) Corn on the cob or sweetcorn (fresh) Cooled samp Cooled mealie meal ROOT VEGETABLES Sweet potato	CITRUS FRUIT All fresh and dried, e.g. oranges, naartjies, limes, grapefruit and lemons DECIDUOUS FRUIT AND BERRIES All fresh and dried e.g. apricots, cherries, peaches, plums, pears, apples, kiwi fruit and grapes – watch portions! CANNED FRUIT All of the above, in fruit juice Pie apples FRUIT JUICE Watch portions! Only 125ml (½ c) at a time, e.g. apple juice, fresh grape-fruit juice, Mango-orange, Mysteries of the Mountain, Secrets of the Valley, Tangerine Teaser PURE FRUIT BARS Trufruco dried fruit bars (Trufruit) Safari Just Fruit bars	All vegetables, except those listed as intermediate or high GI	SUGARS (NB. Overconsump-tion of any of these can lead to gastric discomfort!) Inulin (Fructo-Oligo-Saccharides) and Frutafit (oligo-fructose) Litesse (ultra-refined polydextrose) Sugalite Raffinose Stachyose Galacto-Oligo-Saccharides Pyrodextrins Lactitol Xylitol Isomalt Maltitol Sorbitol Mannitol Fructose Lactose SNACKS Instant pudding made with low-fat or fat-free milk Fine Form Green Fig bar Popcorn (low fat home-made) Sugar-free sweets (that do not contain glucose, dextrose, maltose or malto-dextrin) JAMS Naturlite fruit spreads Fine Form jam	Sugar-free cold drinks Aquellé Lite (flavoured mineral water) Lipton Ice Tea Lite (peach flavour) Biozest Vitrace Ensure Sustagen Glucerna SR Diet Max made with skimmed milk Mageu No1

Intermediate GI (56–69)

Dairy	Cereals and porridges	Starches	Fruit	Vegetables	Sugars and snacks	Drinks
MILK Condensed milk (low-fat) Ice cream Mega Lite	PORRIDGES Oats, raw and cooked (Bokomo, Pick 'n Pay No Name, Spar, Woolworths) Mealie meal porridge, reheated or with added corn CEREALS Strawberry Pops Hunny B's ProNutro Flakes Tastee wheat Maximize Corn Pops Frosties Coco Pops Crunches All Bran Flakes Shredded Wheat	Mealie meal, reheated or with added corn Sweetcorn, cream-style, canned Potatoes: baby or new, in jackets Basmati rice Couscous Samp & beans BREADS Pita Rye (wheat free) CRACKERS Ryvita Crackermates Lites (sesame and poppyseed, and whole-wheat)	TROPICAL FRUIT All fresh and dried, e.g. banana, mango, pawpaw, pineapple, litchi DRIED FRUIT sultanas, dates, raisins CANNED FRUIT Pineapple (canned in syrup or fruit juice) Peaches, apricots, etc. (canned in syrup) FRUIT JUICE Most fruit juices, except those listed as high or low e.g. Apricot, Mango, Orange, Peach, Grapefruit, etc	Beetroot Marog Spinach	SUGARS Sugar or sucrose Invert sugar SNACKS Homewheat Digestive biscuits (Bettasnack) Low-fat biscuits containing oats or oat bran Muffins, low-fat bran and/or fruit Pancakes/crumpets, low-fat containing oats or oat bran Jelly Bokomo Bran & Raisin Bar JAM Jam, home-made with at least 50% fruit Honey, raw	Regular cold drink, cordials and soft drinks

High GI (70+)

Dairy	Cereals and porridges	Starches	Fruit	Vegetables	Sugars and snacks	Drinks
None	Weet Bix (regular & sugar-free) Toasted Muesli Bran (Kellogg's) Caramel Coco Pops Puffed wheat Crunchy Nut Cornflakes ProNutro (flavoured) Rice Crispies Honey O's Nutrific Coco Pops Cornflakes Fruit Loops Special K (Kellogg's) Cooked oat bran Jungle & Tiger Oats Instant Oats Maltabella Mealie meal, refined and coarse Polenta	Instant noodles Pasta, home-made or made from flour or soft SA wheat Millet Potatoes, boiled, mashed, baked and fried Samp Mealie rice 'Sticky' white rice BREADS SA brown, white and regular whole-wheat bread Bread rolls and anything made with cake flour, bread flour, whole-wheat flour, cornflour, rice or potato flour Soup powder or gravy powder Muffins and scones CRACKERS Cream crackers Snack bread (white and whole-wheat) Rice cakes and rice crackers Corn Thins	Melons 'Spanspek' and sweet melon Watermelon Dried fruit Dried fruit rolls FRUIT JUICES Litchi Medley of Fruits	Pumpkin, e.g. Hubbard squash, Butternut and flat, 'boer' pumpkin Carrots Green beans with potato Turnips Parsnips	SUGARS Glucose Dextrose Maltotriose Maltose Maltodextrin SNACKS Marie biscuits, Cream crackers, Boudoir biscuits Cakes Energy Bar, strawberry PVM Tapioca boiled with milk Honey, commercial Boiled and jelly-type sweets	SPORTS DRINKS Game Energade Lucozade Powerade Lucozade-Sport

Breakfast scones

Makes 10 scones

375 ml (1½ c) flour
10 ml (2 t) baking powder
5 ml (1 t) bicarbonate of soda
1 ml (¼ t) salt
60 g oat bran*, pressed down (125 ml [½ cup])
1 medium apple, cored and grated
60 ml (4 T) sultanas or 8 dried apricot halves
45 ml (3 T) soft 'lite' margarine*
1 egg, beaten
125 ml (½ c) skimmed (fat-free) milk* or low-fat
   evaporated milk, chilled and beaten for a lighter
   scone

Nutrients per scone

Glycaemic Index 62 • Carbohydrates 22 g •
Protein 4 g • Fat 3 g • Fibre 2 g • kJ 571 •
Glycaemic load 14

ONE SCONE IS EQUIVALENT TO
1 STARCH + 1 FRUIT + ½ FAT

1 Preheat the oven to 200 °C.
2 Sift the flour, baking powder, bicarbonate of soda and salt together in a large mixing bowl.
3 Add the oat bran and lift a few times with a tablespoon to incorporate air; add the grated apple and sultanas or apricots and mix through.
4 Melt the margarine in the microwave for 20–30 seconds on high. Add the beaten egg and milk and stir. Add to the dry ingredients and stir gently with a fork until a dough forms. Do not overmix.
5 Spoon the dough onto a lightly greased muffin pan.
6 Bake for 15–18 minutes, or until they are golden brown, have risen well and a skewer inserted in the centre comes out clean.

Dietician's notes

- This is a lovely lower fat, lower GI and higher fibre scone than traditional scones, which will neither leave you feeling hungry an hour later, nor add centimetres to your hips.
- These scones can also be served for morning tea or afternoon coffee.
- The dough also makes a good pizza base. Omit the sultanas or dried apricots and use less milk, so that the dough can be handled easily. Omitting the sultanas will raise the GI, but the dough will still have a lower GI than ordinary pizza dough.

Breakfast bars

Makes 15 bars

125 ml (½ c) cake flour
2 ml (½ t) salt
125 ml (½ c) oat bran*
125 ml (½ c) whole-wheat ProNutro*
125 ml (½ c) high-fibre cereal*, crushed
250 ml (1 c) lower GI oats*
1 apple, peeled and grated
125 ml (½ c) sultanas
1 egg white
75 ml (5 T) low-fat fruit yoghurt*
60 ml (4 T) soft 'lite' margarine*
90 ml (6 T) caramel brown sugar
30 ml (2 T) golden syrup
2 ml (½ t) bicarbonate of soda

Nutrients per 50 g bar

Glycaemic Index 59 • Carbohydrates 23 g •
Protein 3 g • Fat 3 g • Fibre 3 g •
kJ 584 • Glycaemic load 14

ONE BREAKFAST BAR IS EQUIVALENT TO
1 STARCH + 1 FRUIT + ½ FAT

1 Preheat the oven to 180 °C.
2 Sift the flour and salt into a large bowl. Add the oat bran, ProNutro, cereal and oats. Lift up with a spoon to aerate.
3 Add the grated apple, sultanas, egg white and yoghurt and mix well.
4 Heat the margarine, sugar and syrup together in a saucepan, stirring until melted. Remove from the heat. Add the bicarbonate of soda, stirring until it foams. Pour over the dry ingredients. Mix well, making sure all the dry ingredients are moistened. The dough will seem a little crumbly.
5 Spoon the dough onto a lightly greased swiss-roll pan, and press down smoothly to approximately 1.5 cm thick, using only half the pan.
6 Bake for 25–30 minutes, or until the breakfast bars are golden brown.
7 Cut into 15 breakfast bars while still warm, using a warm knife.
8 Leave to cool on a cooling rack.

These bars are well worth the effort of making, to have a breakfast-on-the-run available when you need it, or as a sustaining snack before going to gym.

As these bars are quite moist, they do not keep long. Store in an airtight container and freeze them if they have not been eaten within 2 days.

Dietician's notes

- Remember to have at least one glass of liquid when eating these breakfast bars as they contain appreciable quantities of fibre that needs to be hydrated.
- Ideally, you should have some source of protein with this breakfast bar (e.g. a small tub of yoghurt or a hard-boiled egg) to make a complete breakfast.

See page 123 for recipe of Healthy breakfast smoothie pictured opposite.

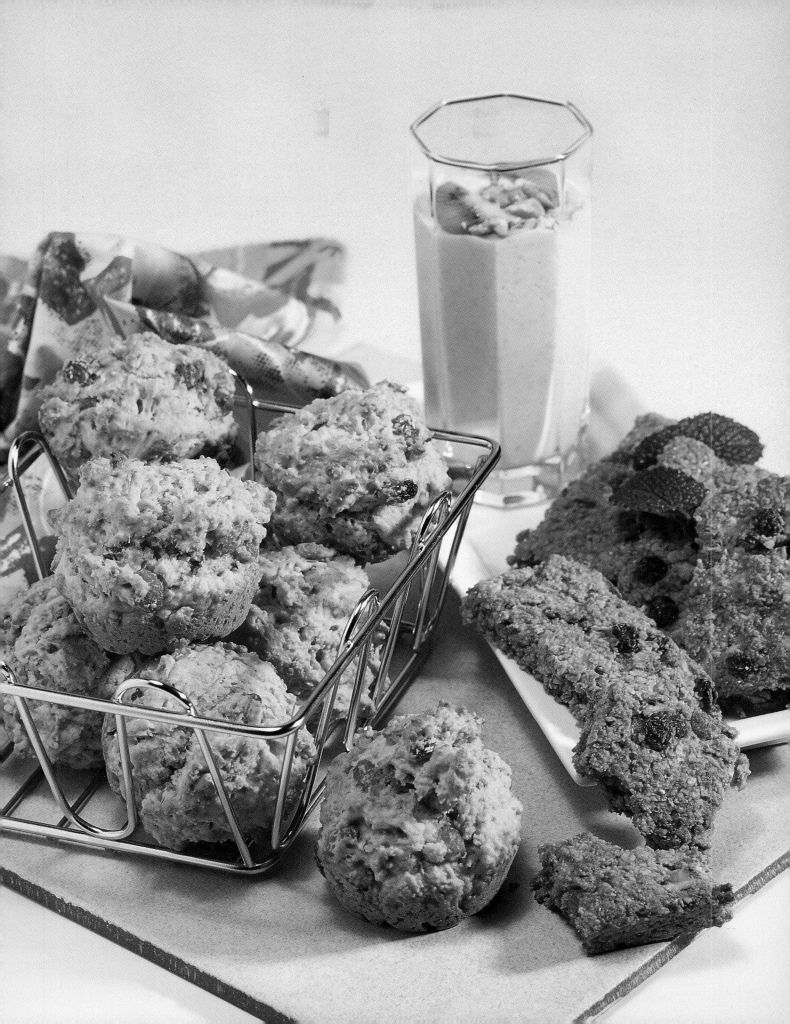

Mozzarella herb muffins
Makes 12 muffins

250 ml (1 c) low-fat buttermilk* or low-fat plain
   yoghurt*
1 egg
15 ml (1 T) olive oil
15 ml (1 T) balsamic vinegar
1 tomato, chopped
1 onion, peeled and chopped
1 clove garlic, chopped or 2 ml (½ t) dried garlic flakes
315 ml (1¼c) flour
12.5 ml (2½ t) baking powder
5 ml (1 t) salt
2 ml (½ t) bicarbonate of soda
175 ml (⅔ c) oat bran*
60 ml (4 T) chopped fresh basil or 5 ml (1 t) dried basil
45 ml (3 T) fresh origanum or 5 ml (1 t) dried origanum
freshly ground black pepper
250 ml (1 c) grated mozzarella (100 g)*

Nutrients per muffin

Glycaemic Index 55 • Carbohydrates 15 g •
Protein 5 g • Fat 4 g • Fibre 2 g • kJ 511 •
Glycaemic load 8

ONE MUFFIN IS EQUIVALENT TO
1 STARCH + ½ DAIRY/MILK

1 Preheat the oven to 200 °C.
2 Mix the buttermilk or yoghurt, egg, oil, vinegar, tomato, onion and garlic in a large measuring jug.
3 Sift the flour, baking powder, salt and bicarbonate of soda into a large bowl. Add the oat bran, basil, origanum, pepper and ¾ of the cheese, and lift up a few times to incorporate air.
4 Pour the yoghurt mixture into the flour mixture and stir until all the ingredients are well mixed.
5 Spoon into a greased muffin pan, overfilling each muffin hollow slightly.
6 Top each muffin with 5 ml (1 t) of the remaining grated cheese.
7 Bake for 25 minutes. Turn off the oven and leave for another 10 minutes.

These savoury muffins make a delicious treat for that special brunch, or for bringing to school functions when you have to supply some eats for tea.
   If possible, use fresh herbs, as they add much more flavour to the muffins.

Dietician's notes
- Note that we used ⅔ flour and ⅓ oat bran (315 ml [1¼ c] flour + 175 ml [⅔ c] oat bran). This ratio of flour and oat bran works well in most muffin recipes.
- The high GI of the flour is offset by adding the yoghurt, onion, tomato and oat bran (all lower GI ingredients), and the result is a lower GI, lower fat muffin.
- These muffins have a low glycaemic load. Most muffins have a glycaemic load of well over 12.
- This is a good alternative to those tempting high-GI, high-fat cheese rolls!

Sweetcorn fritters
Makes 15 fritters

1 x 410 g can creamstyle sweetcorn
80 ml (scant ⅓ c) flour
10 ml (2 t) baking powder
80 ml (scant ⅓ c) oat bran*, pressed down
1 egg, beaten
5 ml (1 t) canola oil for frying

Nutrients per fritter

Glycaemic Index 61 • Carbohydrates 8 g •
Protein 2 g • Fat 1 g • kJ 196 • Fibre 1 g •
Glycaemic load 5

ONE FRITTER IS EQUIVALENT TO
½ STARCH

1 Place the sweetcorn in a mixing bowl.
2 Sift the flour and baking powder over the sweetcorn, add the oat bran and egg, and stir to mix.
3 Heat 5 ml (1 t) oil in a nonstick frying pan. When heated, swirl the oil around and pour out all the excess oil.
4 Drop heaped tablespoonsful of the batter into the pan and fry the fritters on both sides without adding any more oil, until all the batter has been used up. (This is called 'fake' frying.)

Dietician's notes
- This is a tasty lower GI alternative to regular flapjacks and is just as delicious.
- Note that all the batter can be 'fake-fried' in only 5 ml (1 t) oil, which is used to grease the frying pan.
- It is not necessary to spread these fritters with margarine. Eat them dry with a little low GI jam and lower fat cheese, if desired.
- These fritters can also be used as the starch with meat and vegetables.

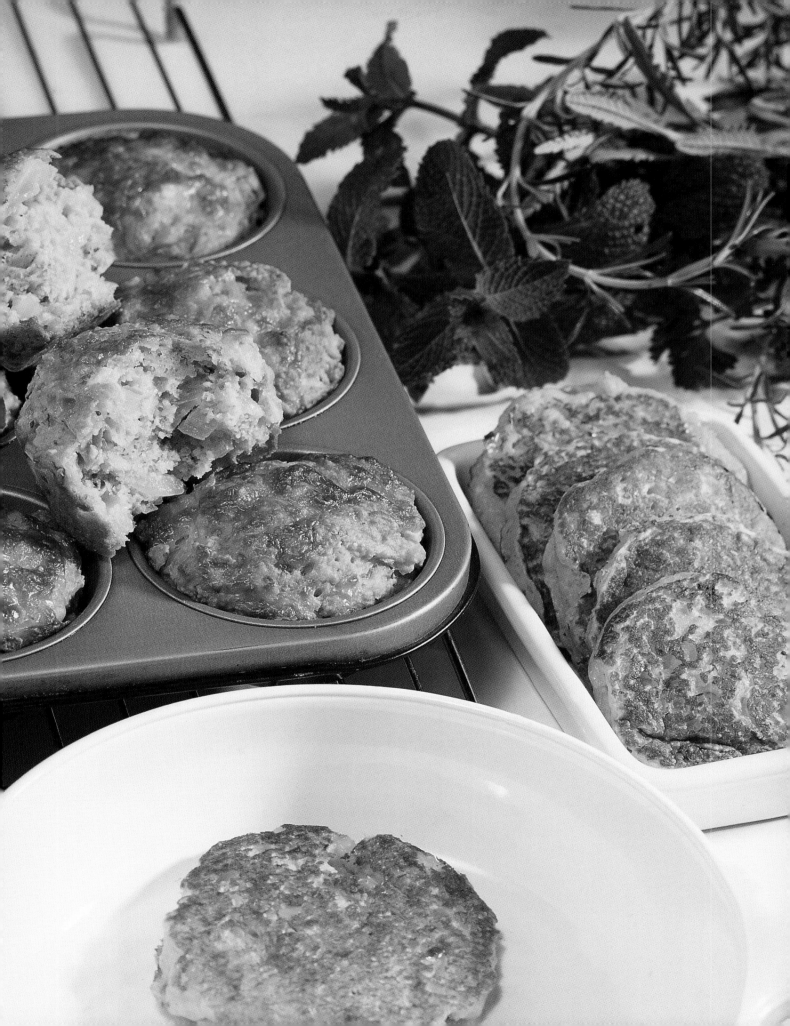

Swiss muesli

Serves 2

125 ml (½ c) lower GI oats* (raw)
175 ml tub low-fat or fat-free fruit yoghurt*,
   sweetened
1 apple, washed (preferably Golden Delicious
   or Starking)
1 medium banana
5 ml (1 t) lemon juice
30 ml (2 T) chopped nuts of your preference

Nutrients per serving

Glycaemic Index 44 • Carbohydrates 49 g •
Protein 10 g • Fat 9 g • Fibre 5 g • kJ 1 318 •
Glycaemic load 22

ONE SERVING IS EQUIVALENT TO
1 STARCH + 1 DAIRY + 1 FRUIT + 1 FAT

1   Mix the oats with the yoghurt.
2   Grate the apple and slice the banana on top of the oat mixture.
3   Pour the lemon juice over and stir well, to prevent discoloration of the fruit.
4   Allow to stand for a while or overnight, if desired.
5   Dish into 2 breakfast bowls and top with the nuts.
6   Serve and enjoy.

You must use sweetened fruit yoghurt, otherwise the muesli will be very sour, due to the presence of the lemon juice.

For a more tart muesli, use yoghurt such as strawberry, youngberry or apricot; for a sweeter muesli, use pear, banana or vanilla yoghurt.

For a roasted muesli taste, place the oats in a roasting pan and roast under the grill for a few minutes, stirring frequently. Allow to cool before making the muesli.

Variation: Layer the oats, yoghurt and fruit in a glass and top with the nuts.

Dietician's notes

• Low-fat or fat-free milk can be used in place of the yoghurt.

Ursula's breakfast muffins

Makes 15 large muffins

125 ml (½ c) oat bran*
125 ml (½ c) whole-wheat flour (Nutty Wheat)
125 ml (½ c) whole-wheat ProNutro*
125 ml (½ c) lower GI oats*
125 ml (½ c) high-fibre cereal*
125 ml (½ c) cake flour
250 ml (1 c) digestive bran (wheat bran)
2 ml (½ t) salt
5 ml (1 t) baking powder
7 ml (1½ t) bicarbonate of soda
125 ml (½ c) sultanas
1 small Granny Smith apple or firm pear, grated
1 small raw sweet potato, grated
1 egg, separated + 1 egg white
5 ml (1 t) vanilla essence
30 ml (2 T) canola oil
125 ml (½ c) soft brown sugar
375 ml (1½ c) fat-free milk

Nutrients per muffin

Glycaemic Index 56 • Carbohydrates 25 g •
Protein 5 g • Fat 3 g • Fibre 5 g • kJ 641 •
Glycaemic load 14

ONE MUFFIN IS EQUIVALENT TO
1½ STARCH + ½ FAT

1   Preheat the oven to 220 °C.
2   Mix all the dry ingredients, then add the sultanas, the grated apple or pear and the sweet potato. Mix gently and set aside.
3   Beat the egg yolk, vanilla essence, oil and sugar together in a large bowl.
4   Add the dry ingredients, alternating with the milk. Mix gently, but thoroughly.
5   Whisk both egg whites to the soft peak stage and gently fold into the batter.
6   Spoon the batter into greased muffin pans, slightly overfilling each muffin hollow, and place in the hot oven.
7   Turn the oven temperature down to 180 °C and bake for 20–25 minutes.
8   Insert a skewer in the centre of a muffin to check whether they are cooked. If there is any raw batter on the skewer, bake for another 5 minutes.

Eat the muffins on the same day, as they do not keep well because of their high moisture content; alternatively, freeze and defrost them individually as needed.

Dietician's notes

• These muffins are particularly high in fibre; good for a healthy bowel, lowering cholesterol levels and lowering blood glucose levels and insulin response.
• Plain flour can be used instead of whole-wheat flour if you prefer less bran in muffins. The GI is the same for both flours.

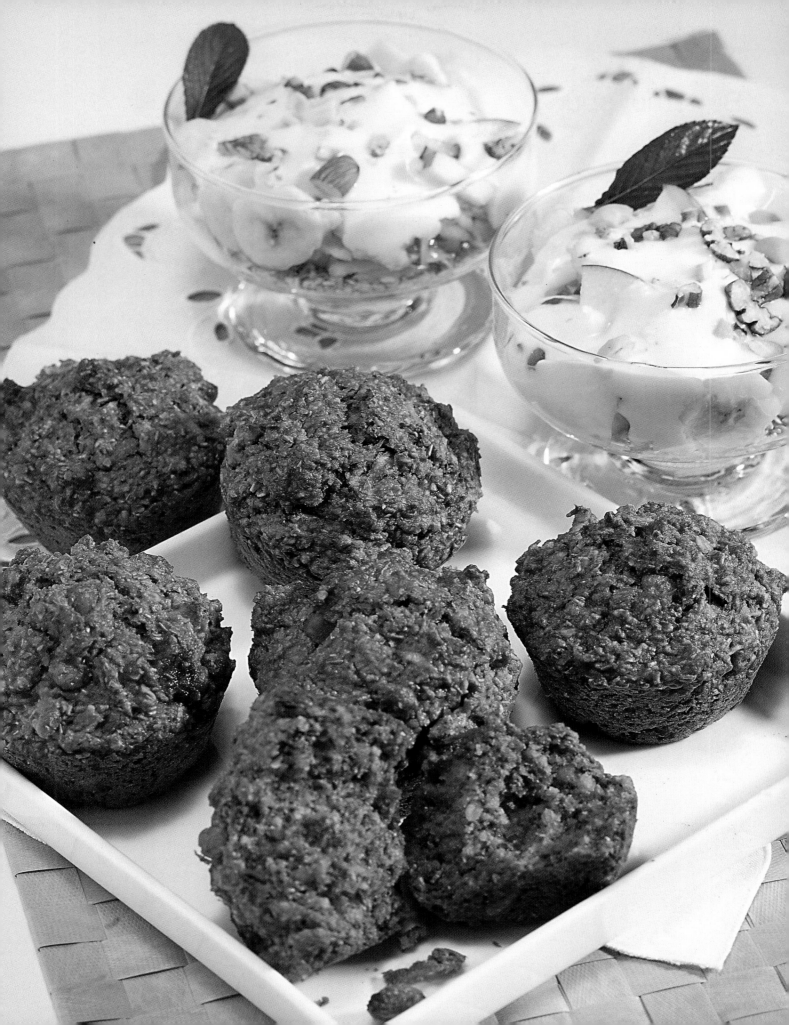

Butternut soup

Serves 10

500 ml (2 c) hot chicken stock (use 2 stock cubes
    and 500 ml [2 c] boiling water)
500 ml (2 c) water
1 kg (2 medium) butternut, peeled and cubed
500 g (1 large) sweet potato, peeled and cubed
2 large green apples, peeled and grated
1 large onion, peeled and finely chopped
185 ml (¾ c) split red lentils*
5 ml (1 t) curry powder
1 large orange
150 ml (⅗ c) low-fat plain yoghurt*
grated nutmeg

1   Pour the chicken stock and water into a very large saucepan.
2   Add the butternut, sweet potato, green apples, onion, lentils and curry powder
    to the stock and water and cook until tender, about 1 hour.
3   Meanwhile, peel the skin off ½ the washed orange (or grate the orange peel) and
    then squeeze out the juice. Set both aside.
4   Cool the soup slightly and then purée it to the desired consistency with the
    orange juice, adding a little milk if it is too thick.
5   Pour the soup back into the saucepan and add the orange peel, then heat through
    gently. Add water if the soup is still too thick.
6   Serve in heated soup bowls with a swirl of yoghurt (15 ml [1 T] per serving) and
    a sprinkling of grated nutmeg.

*This recipe makes a double batch of soup (enough for 10 people). Should you wish
to make only half the recipe, simply halve all the ingredients. If you halve the recipe,
you will only have to cook the soup for 35 minutes before liquidising it.*

Some children won't like the strong taste of orange peel in the soup. Simply omit.

Dietician's notes

*   As we suspect that butternut has a high GI (it has not yet been tested in SA), it is
    important to make sure that you add the lentils, apples and at least half as much
    sweet potato as butternut to offset the higher GI of the butternut.
*   Note the very high fibre content per portion, and that this soup is virtually fat free.
    This means you could enjoy a higher fat pudding (e.g. a bought apple crumble)
    after this soup as your main meal.

Nutrients per serving

Glycaemic Index 47 • Carbohydrates 32 g •
Protein 8 g • Fat 1 g • Fibre 8 g • kJ 705 •
Glycaemic load 15

ONE SERVING OF SOUP IS EQUIVALENT TO
1 STARCH + 1 PROTEIN + 1 VEGETABLE

Hearty winter soup

Serves 4

5 ml (1 t) oil*
1 medium onion, peeled and finely chopped
5 ml (1 t) dried garlic flakes or crushed garlic
    or 1 clove garlic, finely chopped
2 pieces soup meat, cubed and fat discarded
    (500 g with bone)
10 ml (2 t) beef stock powder or ½ beef stock cube
5 ml (1 t) dried rosemary
1 ml (¼ t) ground cloves
1 large carrot, peeled and grated
1 baby marrow, trimmed and grated
1 celery stalk, sliced
1 leek, sliced
1.5 litres (6 c) water
60 g (⅓ c) soup mix* or split lentils*

1   Heat the oil and fry the onion and garlic until the onion is transparent.
2   Add the meat (including the bones), the stock powder or crumbled cube, and the
    rosemary and cloves, and fry for a few minutes.
3   Add the carrot, baby marrow, celery and leek.
4   Add the water and soup mix or split lentils, stir and then boil for about 1 hour, or
    until the soup has thickened.
5   Serve with 1–2 slices of seed loaf per person.

*If you prefer to use fresh rosemary, add more than the dried quantity and add it
towards the end of the cooking process. Dried herbs, however, have to be added at
the start of cooking, to allow the flavour to penetrate the dish.*

Dietician's notes

*   Its low GL and exceptionally high fibre content make this delicious soup a really
    good choice.
*   Please note that, in spite of the higher GI carrot in the soup, this soup is still low
    GI, as there are enough other low GI ingredients to counteract the high GI of the
    carrots. Carrots also have a low GL, as they contain very little carbohydrate.

Nutrients per serving

Glycaemic Index <40 • Carbohydrates 28 g •
Protein 28 g • Fat 9 g • Fibre 7 g • kJ 1 415 •
Glycaemic load 10

ONE SERVING OF SOUP IS EQUIVALENT TO
1½ STARCH + 3 PROTEIN + 1 VEGETABLE

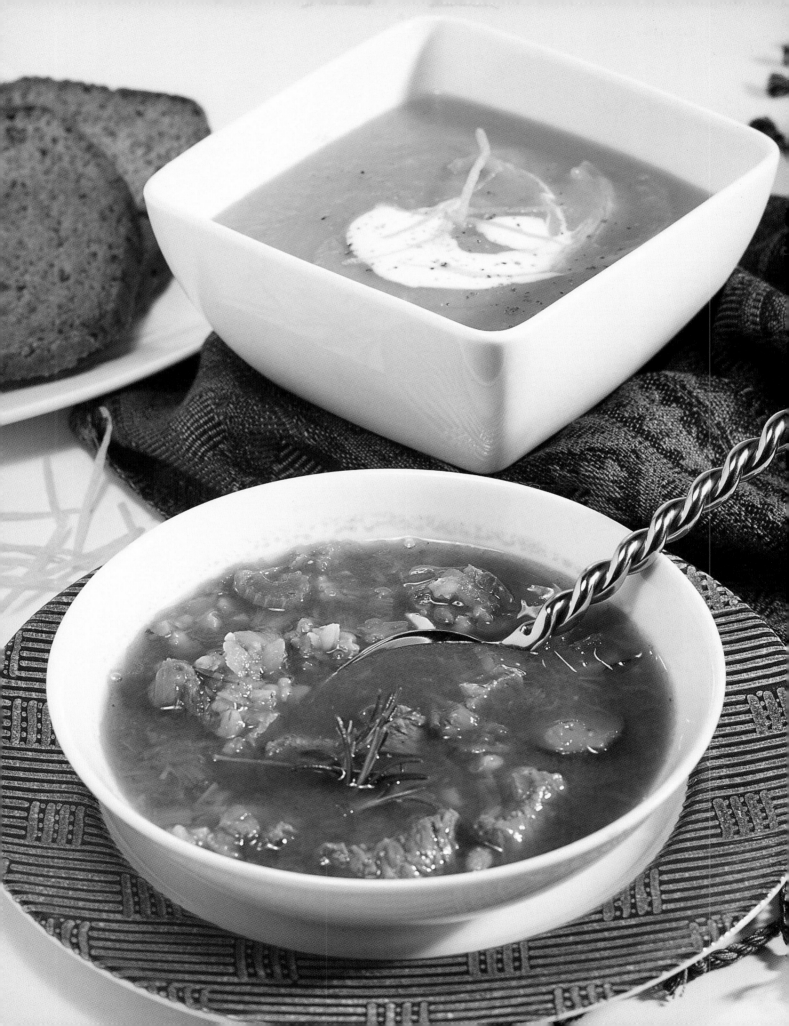

Bean soup

Serves 4

5 ml (1 t) oil

1 medium onion, peeled and finely chopped

60 g bacon* (4 rashers), chopped and fat discarded

2 x 410 g cans sugar beans* or 500 ml (2 c) cooked
   dry beans

500 ml (2 c) water

5 ml (1 t) salt

ground pepper to taste

60 ml (4 T) lower GI oats*

250 ml (1 c) fat-free or low-fat milk*

125 ml (½ c) chopped fresh basil leaves
   or 10 ml (2 t) dried sweet basil

15 ml (1 T) lemon juice

Nutrients per serving

Glycaemic Index <40 • Carbohydrates 34 g •
Protein 15 g • Fat 5 g • Fibre 11 g • kJ 1 153 •
Glycaemic load 9

ONE SERVING OF SOUP IS EQUIVALENT TO
2 STARCH + 2 LEAN PROTEIN

1   Heat the oil in a saucepan and fry the onion until transparent.
2   Add the bacon and fry until crisp.
3   Add the canned beans with their liquid (or the cooked beans with a little extra water), as well as the extra 500 ml (2 c) water.
4   Boil, covered, for 30 minutes.
5   Mash the beans, add salt and pepper and boil for another 15 minutes.
6   Add the oats, milk and basil and boil for another 15 minutes.
7   Lastly, add the lemon juice.
8   Serve as a light meal, on its own or with 1 slice lower GI Health bread (page 96) and a little lower fat cheese, if desired.

Make this soup the day before and simply reheat for a delicious, filling, quick lunch on a cold winter's day.

Dietician's notes

• The lemon juice helps to bring out the flavour of the bean soup and lowers the GI even further.
• The nutritional analysis was done with fat-free milk. The fat content will be slightly higher if low-fat milk is used.
• Note the exceptionally high fibre content and the low Glycaemic load for this filling soup.

Quick 'n easy minestrone soup

Serves 4

5 ml (1 t) olive or canola oil

1 onion, peeled and finely chopped

2 cloves garlic, minced

1 carrot, grated

1 celery stalk, chopped

250 ml (1 c) broccoli florets, chopped

1.5 litres (6 c) chicken stock (make with 20 ml [4 t]
   chicken stock powder and 1.5 litres [6 c] hot water)

1 x 410 g can baked beans in tomato sauce*

100 g dry spaghetti*, broken into 2 cm lengths
   (250 ml [1 c])

10 ml (2 t) dried mixed herbs

100 ml (⅖ c) chopped fresh parsley

Nutrients per serving

Glycaemic Index 44 • Carbohydrates 43 g •
Protein 10 g • Fat 3 g • Fibre 10 g • kJ 971 •
Glycaemic load 19

ONE SERVING IS EQUIVALENT TO
2 STARCH + 1 PROTEIN + VEGETABLES

1   Heat the oil and gently fry the onion and garlic until the onion is transparent.
2   Add the carrot and celery, and stir-fry for 3 minutes.
3   Add the broccoli and toss all the ingredients together.
4   Pour the stock over the vegetables and simmer for 10 minutes.
5   Add the baked beans and bring the soup back to the boil.
6   Add the broken spaghetti and herbs and simmer for 10 minutes, or until the pasta is just soft.
7   Sprinkle with chopped fresh parsley and serve.

Dietician's notes

• This soup makes a meal on its own for lunch on a cold day.
• The baked beans add loads of typical tomato flavour and keep blood glucose levels steady for at least 3 hours.
• Should you wish to eat a slice of lower GI Health bread (page 96) with this soup, have a smaller portion of the soup.

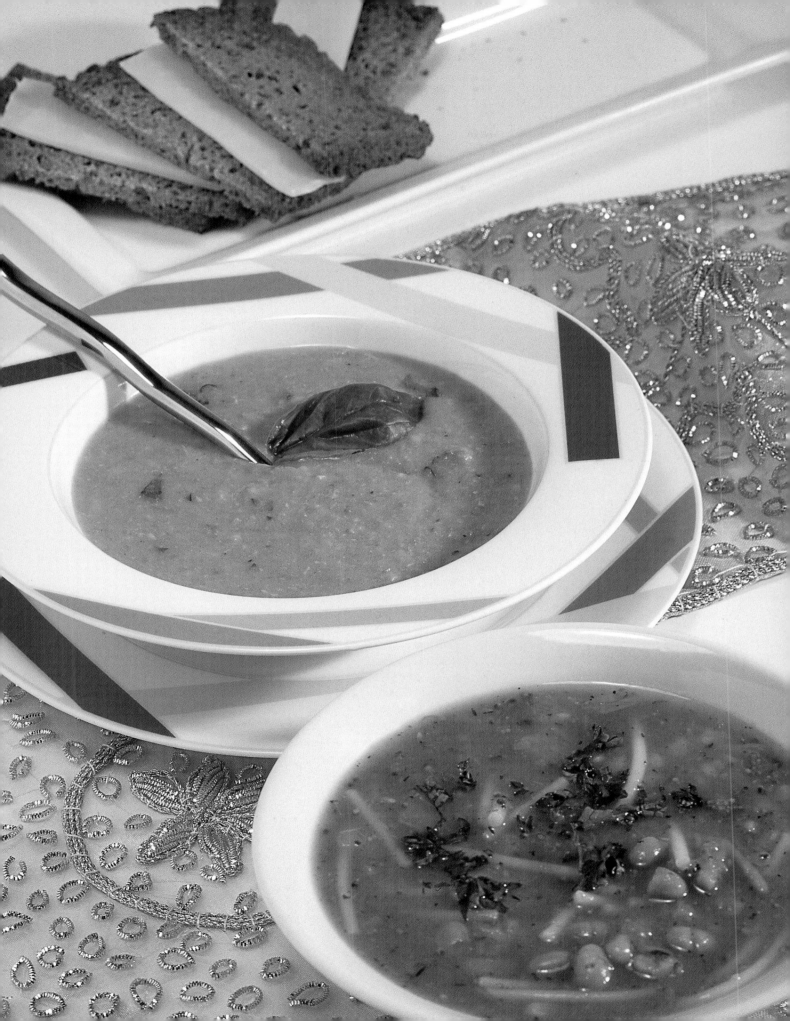

Cucumber salad

Serves 4

1 English cucumber
DRESSING
5 ml (1 t) olive oil
1 spring onion, chopped
2 ml (½ t) ground ginger
2 ml (½ t) ground cinnamon
2 ml (½ t) ground coriander
2 ml (½ t) turmeric
15 ml (1 T) soy sauce
60 ml (4 T) low-fat plain yoghurt*
1 gherkin, chopped
30 ml (2 T) freshly squeezed lemon juice
    (about ½ lemon)
5 ml (1 t) raw honey

1 Quarter the whole cucumber lengthways and slice thinly into a salad bowl.
2 Heat the oil in a small saucepan and gently fry the spring onion and the spices
    for 3 minutes to develop the spice flavours. Spoon into a small mixing bowl.
3 Add the rest of the ingredients for the dressing, and mix gently.
4 Pour over the sliced cucumber in the salad bowl.
5 Allow to stand for 1 hour before serving.

A deliciously different cucumber salad, with an Asian touch.

Dietician's note

*   Cucumbers (and this cucumber salad) have a very low GI and GL. They are ideal for slimming and generally healthy eating habits, as they stimulate the metabolism and help to add bulk to the meal, without adding too many kilojoules or fat.

Nutrients per serving

Glycaemic Index 22 • Carbohydrates 6 g •
Protein 2 g • Fat 1 g • Fibre 1 g • kJ 173 •
Glycaemic load 1

ONE SERVING IS EQUIVALENT TO
1 VEGETABLE

Winter 'salad'

Makes 2 litres (8 c)

5 ml (1 t) oil*
1 medium onion, peeled and chopped finely or grated
1 medium green sweet pepper, chopped finely or
    grated
1 medium red sweet pepper, chopped finely or grated
2 cloves garlic, chopped finely or 5 ml (1 t) dried garlic
    flakes
¼ cabbage, shredded or grated
1 x 400 g can tomatoes, chopped finely
1.5 litres (6 c) boiling water
125 ml (½ c) soup mix* and 10 ml (2 t) vegetable stock
    powder or 1 x 40–50 g packet onion soup powder
5 ml (1 t) dried herbs e.g. sweet basil

1 Heat the oil in a saucepan.
2 Fry the onion, green pepper, red pepper and garlic in the oil until softened.
3 Add the cabbage and stir until well mixed.
4 Add the tomatoes and 1.25 litres (5 c) of the boiling water.
5 Mix the remaining boiling water with the soup mix or onion soup powder and add
    to the soup, together with the dried herbs.
6 Cover and boil for 30 minutes (if soup powder is used) or at least 60 minutes (if
    soup mix is used).
7 Serve instead of salad with light meals.

The soup will have an extra-delicious flavour if canned tomatoes flavoured with herbs are used. They are available in most supermarkets.
    This soup can be eaten as is, or it can be puréed to yield a thick vegetable soup. More water can be added if you want a thinner soup.
    Store the soup in the fridge and simply reheat it in the microwave when needed.

Dietician's notes

*   We specifically included this soup to be used instead of salad in winter, as most people eat salad ingredients with their light meal in summer, and simply omit salad in winter. Eating a cup of this soup in winter will effectively replace a cup of summer salad and will increase the satiety value of the meal.
*   In spite of the fact that soup powder has a high GI value, its GI is effectively lowered in this recipe by all the low GI vegetables.

Nutrients per serving

Glycaemic Index <40 • Carbohydrates 10 g •
Protein 3 g • Fat 1 g • Fibre 3 g • kJ 279 •
Glycaemic load 3

ONE SERVING IS EQUIVALENT TO
2 VEGETABLES

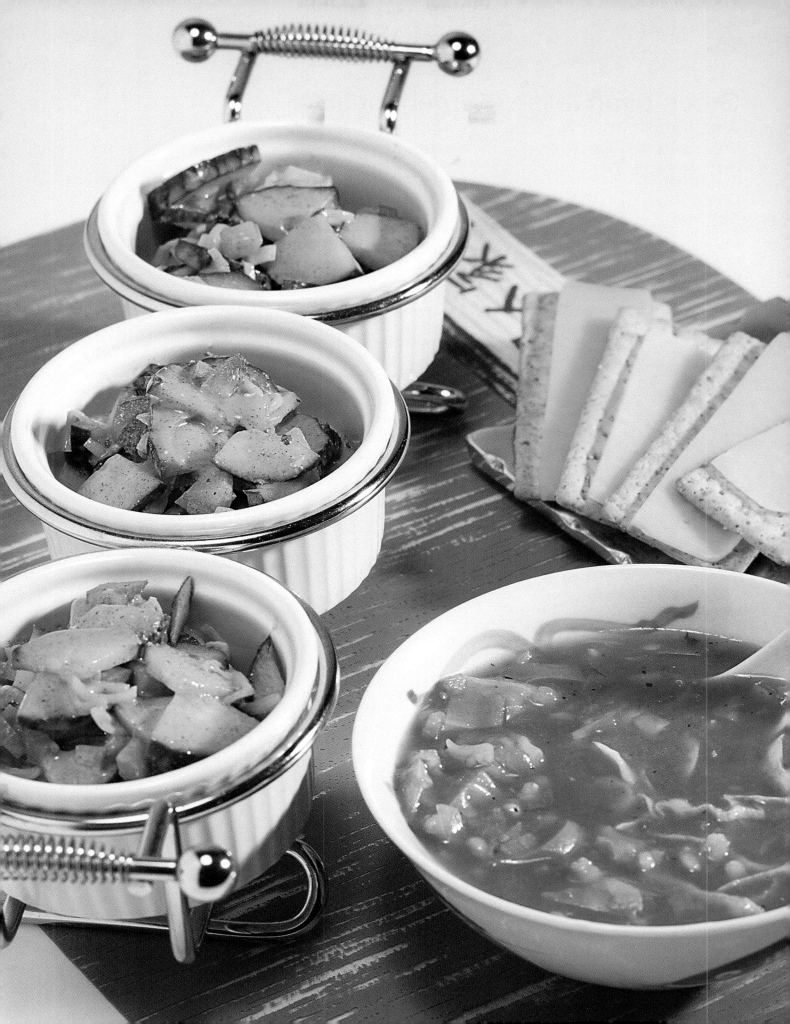

Green bean relish (Kerrieboontjies)

Serves 12   Makes 1 litre (4 c)

500 g fresh green beans, trimmed and sliced
2 large onions, thinly sliced
150 ml (⅗ c) vinegar
5 ml (1 t) salt
60 ml (4 T) sugar
185 ml (scant ¾ c) apple juice*
5 ml (1 t) mustard powder
5 ml (1 t) curry powder
15 ml (1 T) cornflour (e.g. Maizena)
5 ml (1 t) turmeric
25 ml (5 t) water

1 Cook the green beans and onions in 250 ml (1 c) boiling water until tender, about 10 minutes, then drain.
2 Place the vinegar, salt, sugar and apple juice in a very large saucepan, and bring to the boil. Stir to dissolve the sugar.
3 Add the cooked beans and onions and simmer over medium heat for 15 minutes to allow the vegetables to absorb the flavour.
4 Meanwhile, make a paste of the mustard powder, curry powder, cornflour, turmeric and water.
5 Pour the paste slowly into the hot bean relish; stir well and boil until the relish thickens.
6 Spoon the relish into hot, sterilised jars and seal immediately. Store in the fridge for up to 1 month.
7 Serve as a side salad with meals.

The recipe can easily be doubled or trebled, should you wish to make a stock of this handy salad for the summer months. Remember to store the beans in the fridge.

Dietician's notes

- Because of its extreme acidity, vinegar effectively lowers the GI of any dish.
- This relish is suitable for those who suffer from diabetes, despite the sugar and the cornflour, because of the low GI and GL.

Nutrients per serving
(100 g = 125 ml [½ c])
Glycaemic Index 46 • Carbohydrates 12 g • Protein 1 g • Fat negl • Fibre 1 g • kJ 236 • Glycaemic load 6

ONE SERVING IS EQUIVALENT TO 1 LIMITED VEGETABLE OR 1 FRUIT

Waldorf salad with pears

Serves 8 as a side salad, 4 as lunch

4 pears, cored and sliced lengthways (about 140 g each)
30 ml (2 T) freshly squeezed lemon juice (about ½ lemon)
6 pecans or walnuts, halved (20 g)
1 stalk celery, chopped
125 ml (½ c) grapes, halved and pitted or 60 ml (4 T) sultanas
5 dates, chopped
60 ml (4 T) low-fat or fat-free plain yoghurt*
60 ml (4 T) low-fat mayonnaise*
lettuce leaves to serve (optional)

1 Place the pear slices in a salad bowl and pour the lemon juice over. Mix to cover pears well and prevent discoloration.
2 Add the nuts, celery, grapes or sultanas and dates.
3 Mix the yoghurt and mayonnaise together and spoon over the salad. Toss.
4 Chill until needed, and then serve on a bed of lettuce, or in individual bowls as shown opposite.

This is a delicious alternative to a mixed salad.

Dietician's notes

- The quantity of yoghurt can be doubled, if you want more dressing.
- Add 2 chopped cooked chicken breasts to the salad, and you will have a complete meal – no need to add bread.
- If this salad is eaten as a light meal, it will serve 4 women or 2 men.

Nutrients per serving (Side salad)
Glycaemic Index 45 • Carbohydrates 19 g • Protein 1 g • Fat 3 g • Fibre 3 g • kJ 465 • Glycaemic load 9

ONE SERVING AS A SIDE SALAD IS EQUIVALENT TO 1 FRUIT OR 1 LIMITED VEGETABLE + ½ FAT

ONE SERVING AS A LUNCH (WITH CHICKEN) IS EQUIVALENT TO 1 FRUIT OR LIMITED VEGETABLE + 1 STARCH + 2 LEAN PROTEIN

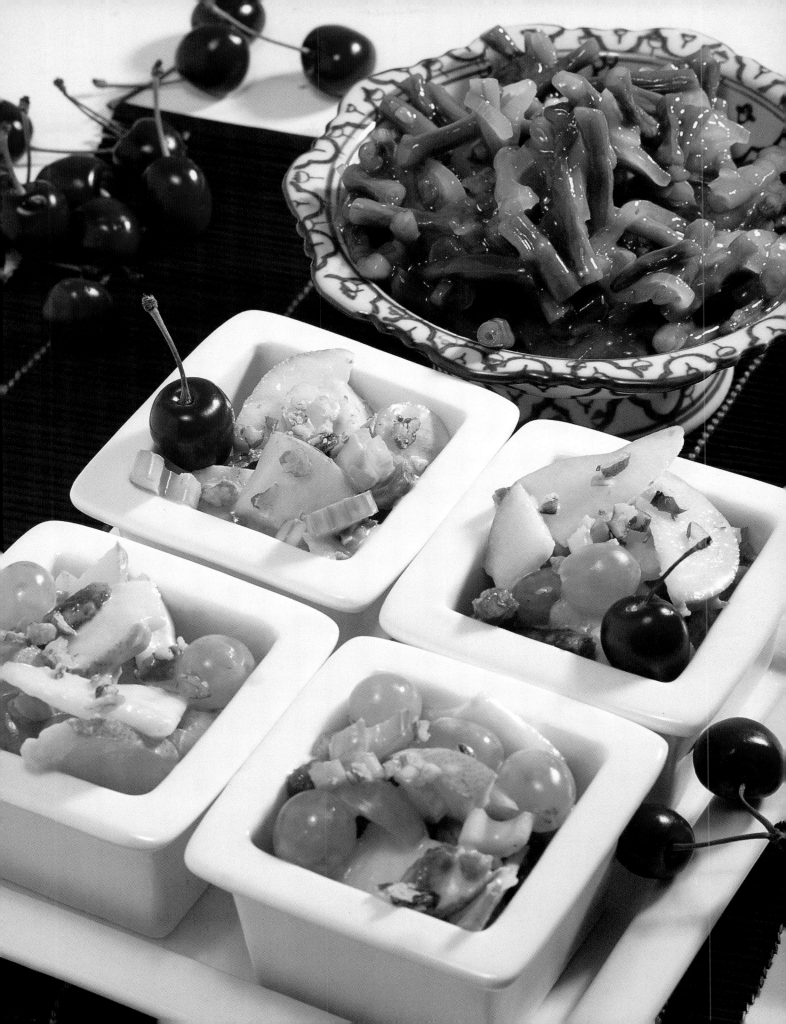

Aurelia's pizzas

Serves 4

4 slices seed loaf or wheat-free rye bread*
1 x 65 g can tomato paste
5 mushrooms, sliced (optional)
1 slice brown bread, crumbled in a food processor
2 ml (½ t) dried garlic flakes
5 (1 t) dried origanum
100 g mozzarella, grated

Nutrients per serving

Glycaemic Index 54 • Carbohydrates 21 g •
Protein 9 g • Fat 7 g • Fibre 3 g • kJ 751 •
Glycaemic load 11

ONE 'PIZZA' IS EQUIVALENT TO
1½ STARCH + 1 PROTEIN

1　Preheat the grill.
2　Lightly toast the bread.
3　Spread tomato paste on the bread.
4　Arrange the sliced mushrooms on the bread.
5　In a medium-sized bowl, mix the breadcrumbs, garlic, origanum and cheese and spread evenly onto the 4 slices of bread.
6　Place the 'pizzas' in an ovenproof dish, sprayed with nonstick spray.
7　Cook directly under the grill for 3 minutes, until the cheese bubbles.

For extra zest, add a little 'lite' chutney, or chillies.

Dietician's notes

- These 'pizzas' are delicious and easy to make – and one of Liesbet's youngest daughter's 'inventions'.
- This grilled dish makes a lovely light lunch or supper, when served with a salad.

Biltong quiche

Serves 8

BASE
250 ml (1 c) flour, sifted before measuring
125 ml (½ c) oat bran*
10 ml (2 t) mustard powder
1 ml (¼ t) salt
45 ml (3 T) soft 'lite' margarine*
1 egg
45 ml (3 T) ice-cold water
FILLING
5 ml (1 t) canola or olive oil*
1 large onion, peeled and chopped
50 g sliced biltong (no fat)
1 x 225 g can baked beans in tomato sauce*, drained
1 egg
1 egg white
125 ml (½ c) skimmed milk*
125 ml (½ c) fat-free or low-fat cottage cheese*
15 ml (1 T) chopped fresh basil
freshly ground black pepper to taste
60 g lower fat cheese*, grated (2 'matchboxes' cheese, before grating)
125 ml (½ cup) grated or powdered biltong (50 g)

Nutrients per serving

Glycaemic Index 56 • Carbohydrates 21 g •
Protein 16 g • Fat 8 g • Fibre 3 g • kJ 939 •
Glycaemic load 12

ONE PORTION OF QUICHE IS EQUIVALENT TO
2 PROTEIN + 1 STARCH

1　Preheat the oven to 200 °C.
2　Spray a quiche pan with nonstick spray.
3　For the base, rub together the flour, oat bran, mustard powder, salt and margarine until the mixture resembles breadcrumbs.
4　Combine the egg and water. Add 15 ml (1 T) egg mixture at a time to the flour mixture and mix to a soft dough. Add more flour if it becomes sticky. Cover with plastic wrap or waxed paper and chill for 20–30 minutes.
5　Press the dough into the quiche pan with your fingers, or roll out the dough and use to line the pan.
6　For the filling, heat the oil in a saucepan and fry the onion. Allow the onion to cool, then spread it evenly over the base of the quiche.
7　Sprinkle the sliced biltong evenly over the onion.
8　Arrange the drained baked beans on top.
9　Beat the whole egg and egg white together. Add the milk, cottage cheese, basil and pepper and mix gently until there are no lumps. Add half of the grated cheese, and mix through.
10　Pour the egg mixture over the quiche, and sprinkle the rest of the grated cheese and the grated or powdered biltong on top.
11　Bake for 15 minutes. Reduce the oven temperature to 180 °C and bake for another 15 minutes, or until set.

This quiche can be frozen, so it is most practical to make two smaller quiches; one for eating and one for freezing.

Dietician's notes

- One eighth of the quiche (1 portion) with a salad of your choice (see pages 34–37) makes a complete meal.
- Please note that the nutritional analysis was made using fat-free cottage cheese. The fat and kJ content will be slightly higher if low-fat cottage cheese is used.

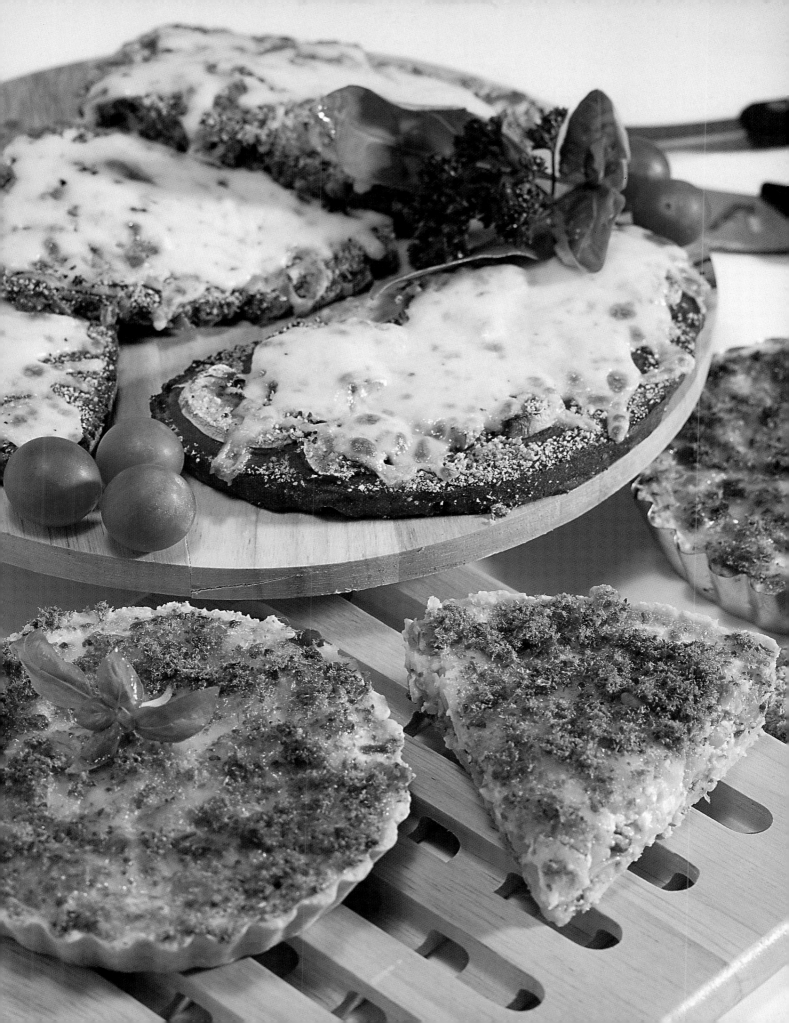

Cold curried chicken mayonnaise

Serves 4

5 ml (1 t) olive/canola oil*

1 onion, peeled and chopped

15 ml (1 T) curry powder

250 ml (1 c) chicken stock or 10 ml (2 t) stock powder
    dissolved in 250 ml (1 c) boiling water

10 ml (2 t) tomato purée

15 ml (1 T) lemon juice

30 ml (2 T) chutney

60 ml (4 T) low-fat 'lite' mayonnaise

200 ml (⅘ c) fat-free plain yoghurt*

400 g chicken breasts (4 medium), skinned, cooked
    and cut into bite-sized pieces

250 ml (1 c) cooked basmati rice*

12 cashew nuts, chopped roughly

Nutrients per serving

Glycaemic Index 40 • Carbohydrates 27 g •
Protein 35 g • Fat 11 g • Fibre 1 g • kJ 1 485 •
Glycaemic load 11

ONE SERVING IS EQUIVALENT TO
1 STARCH + 3 PROTEIN + ½ FAT

1 Heat the oil in a saucepan and stir-fry the onion until transparent.
2 Add the curry powder and cook for 1 minute, stirring continuously.
3 Stir the stock, tomato purée, lemon juice and chutney into the onion mixture and bring to the boil. Reduce the heat and simmer for 5 minutes.
4 Cool the sauce for at least 30 minutes (the sauce can be frozen at this stage).
5 Add the mayonnaise and the yoghurt to the curry mixture and mix well.
6 Add the cooked chicken pieces and rice, and toss lightly.
7 Serve in half a scooped-out pineapple, and sprinkle with the cashew nuts.

Serving this salad in half a scooped-out pineapple looks super special! The pineapple can be cut as pictured, or lengthwise, leaves and all.

Dietician's notes

- Adding some of the fresh pineapple to the salad provides extra zing. Use 50 g chopped pineapple per person. The GI will then rise to 46, which is still low GI and will control blood glucose levels just as effectively as without the pineapple.
- Sweetcorn (whole corn kernels), cooked pasta, barley or wheat rice can be used in place of the rice as they are all low GI starches. Use in the same quantities.
- Note how we have 'diluted' the higher fat mayonnaise with fat-free yoghurt and still produced a deliciously creamy dressing. By doing this, we had some fat units to spare, so to speak, so we could add a few cashew nuts to sprinkle on top and make this a really special salad.

Smoked fish bake

Serves 4

500 g smoked fish e.g. haddock

100 g snoek (optional)

1 onion, peeled and chopped

5 ml (1 t) dried sweet basil

5 ml (1 t) dried mixed herbs

5 ml (1 t) dried parsley

5 ml (1 t) mustard powder

30 ml (2 T) cake flour

375 ml (1½ c) fat-free milk*

2 eggs, beaten

1 egg white

60 g mozzarella*, grated (2 'matchboxes' before
    grating)

Nutrients per serving

(Fish bake and mealie bread)
Glycaemic Index 53 • Carbohydrates 30 g •
Protein 43 g • Fat 11 g • Fibre 3 g • kJ 1 718 •
Glycaemic load 16

ONE PORTION FISH BAKE AND BREAD IS EQUIVALENT TO
4 PROTEIN + 1 STARCH

1 Preheat the oven to 180 °C.
2 Place the fish in a little water and poach for 15 minutes or until cooked.
3 Cool slightly, then remove the bones and flake the fish. In a large bowl, mix the fish, onion, herbs and mustard powder.
4 Sprinkle the flour over the fish and mix gently.
5 Place the milk in another bowl; add the egg and egg white and beat well.
6 Pour the milk and egg mixture over the fish mixture.
7 Mix gently and pour into a greased baking dish.
8 Sprinkle the cheese on top and bake for 45 minutes, or until the dish is set.
9 Serve with 1 slice Mealie bread (page 96) each, fresh from the oven, and a large tossed salad.

Dietician's notes

- Using the 100 g smoked snoek in addition to the 500 g haddock will intensify the flavour. Should you only use haddock, the fat content will drop by 1 g per portion.
- Snoek and haddock are both high in sodium, so do not add any salt to this meal.
- As the fat content is already 11 g for the meal, do not butter the bread, and use lemon juice or balsamic vinegar on the salad, instead of regular dressing.
- The protein content of this meal is higher than that recommended for a light meal. To compensate, therefore, we recommend adding a little carbohydrate, but not too much, such as 1 slice of Mealie bread (see page 96 for the recipe).

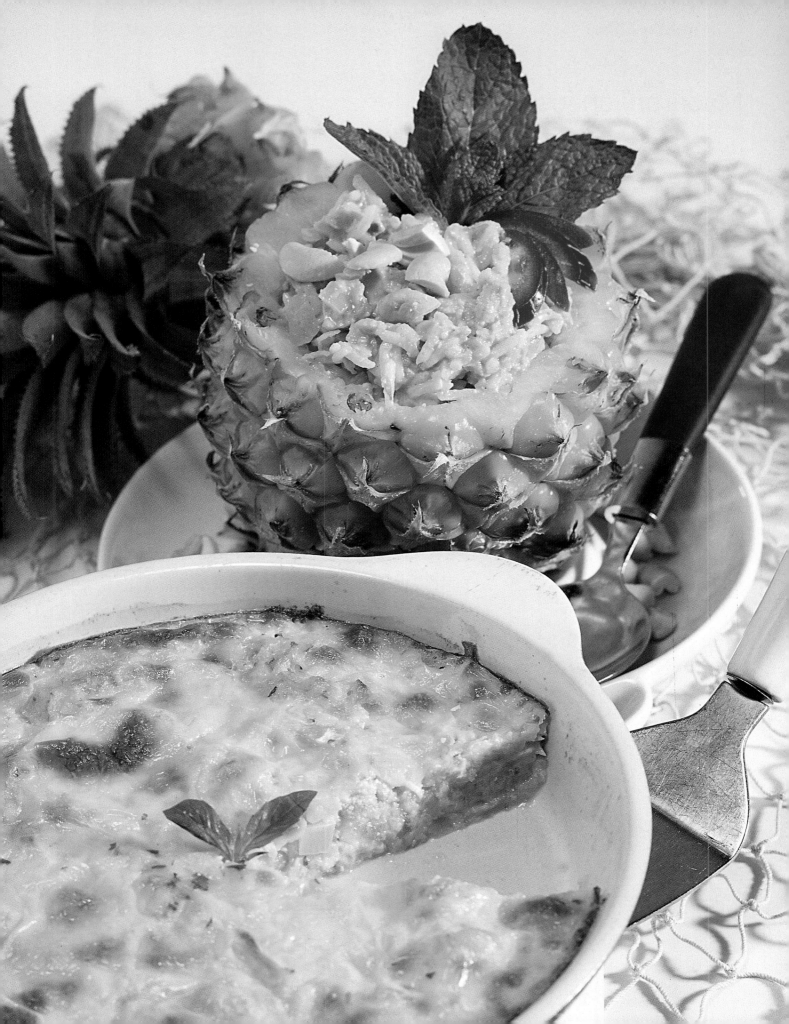

Macaroni cheese

Serves 4

1.5 litres (6 c) boiling water
2 ml (½ t) salt
5 ml (1 t) olive oil*
180 g (6 handfuls or about ⅓ of 500 g packet) uncooked macaroni (durum wheat)*
1 medium onion, peeled and chopped
3 rashers lean bacon*, fat trimmed off, chopped
250 ml (1 c) skimmed milk*
100 ml (⅖ c) vegetable stock or water from cooking vegetables or 5 ml (1t) stock powder dissolved in 100 ml (⅖ c) boiling water
45 ml (3 T) flour
2 ml (½ t) salt
2 ml (½ t) mustard powder
5 ml (1 t) dried mixed herbs
1 tomato, sliced
90 g low-fat mozzarella*, grated

Nutrients per serving

Glycaemic Index 44 • Carbohydrates 52 g • Protein 19 g • Fat 9 g • Fibre 4 g • kJ 1 522 • Glycaemic load 23

ONE SERVING OF MACARONI CHEESE IS EQUIVALENT TO 3 STARCH + 1½ DAIRY/PROTEIN + 1 VEGETABLE

1 In a large saucepan, bring the water, salt and oil to boil.
2 Add the macaroni and boil until just done. Drain cooked pasta and set aside.
3 Preheat the oven to 180 °C. Place the onion and chopped bacon in a dry saucepan and put it on a stove plate.
4 Heat the stove plate to moderate heat and cook without extra oil, stirring continuously. Add a little water if it starts to burn.
5 When the onion is cooked, add the milk and vegetable stock or water, and bring to the boil.
6 In a 500 ml (2 c) glass bowl or jug, mix together the flour, salt, mustard powder and herbs with a little water to make a smooth paste.
7 Pour some of the hot milk from the saucepan onto the flour paste and stir well to ensure there are no lumps.
8 Pour the flour and milk mixture back into the saucepan of hot milk and stir over heat until the sauce thickens.
9 Pour the white sauce over the cooked macaroni, mix gently.
10 Spoon into an ovenproof dish. Decorate with tomato slices and top with cheese.
11 Bake for 30 minutes, or until the cheese is golden brown on top.
12 Serve with a mixed salad for a complete meal.

Dietician's notes

- There is no need to add any extra protein (meat) to this meal.
- If you prefer, omit the mixed salad and serve a fruit salad for dessert. Either will supply the vitamins for the meal.
- The smaller quantity of protein in the meal compensates for the starch.
- For a vegetarian version, leave out the bacon.

Pancakes

Makes 6 pancakes

1 egg
5 ml (1 t) oil e.g. macadamia oil*
1 ml (¼ t) vinegar
185 ml (¾ c) cake flour
1 ml (¼ t) salt
60 ml (4 T) oat bran*, pressed down
250 ml (1 c) fat-free or low-fat milk*
5 ml (1 t) baking powder

Nutrients per pancake

Glycaemic Index 62 • Carbohydrates 16 g • Protein 5 g • Fat 2 g • kJ 447 • Fibre 1 g • Glycaemic load 10

ONE PANCAKE IS EQUIVALENT TO 1 STARCH + ½ FAT

1 Beat together the egg, oil and vinegar, using an electric mixer.
2 In a separate bowl, sift the flour and salt, and add the oat bran. Lift up a few times with a spoon to incorporate air.
3 Add the mixed dry ingredients in 3 batches to the egg and oil mixture, alternating with the milk. Beat after each addition, but not longer than 1 minute at a time.
4 Lastly, add the baking powder and stir in gently.
5 Allow to stand so that the oat bran can hydrate. This yields a better end product. Stir in a little extra milk if the batter is too thick.
6 'Fake fry' (see page 44) in a small to medium-sized nonstick frying pan.
7 Serve with a savoury filling e.g. curried mince and lentils, or a sweet filling such as 5 ml (1 t) cinnamon sugar per pancake, as well as a salad, e.g. Winter 'salad' (page 34).

This recipe can easily be doubled, trebled, etc.

Dietician's notes

- If you suffer from diabetes, 1 savoury pancake and 1 sweet pancake (or 2 for men) will not compromise blood glucose control, especially if the mince mixture contains lentils or beans and if lemon juice is added to the sweet pancake.

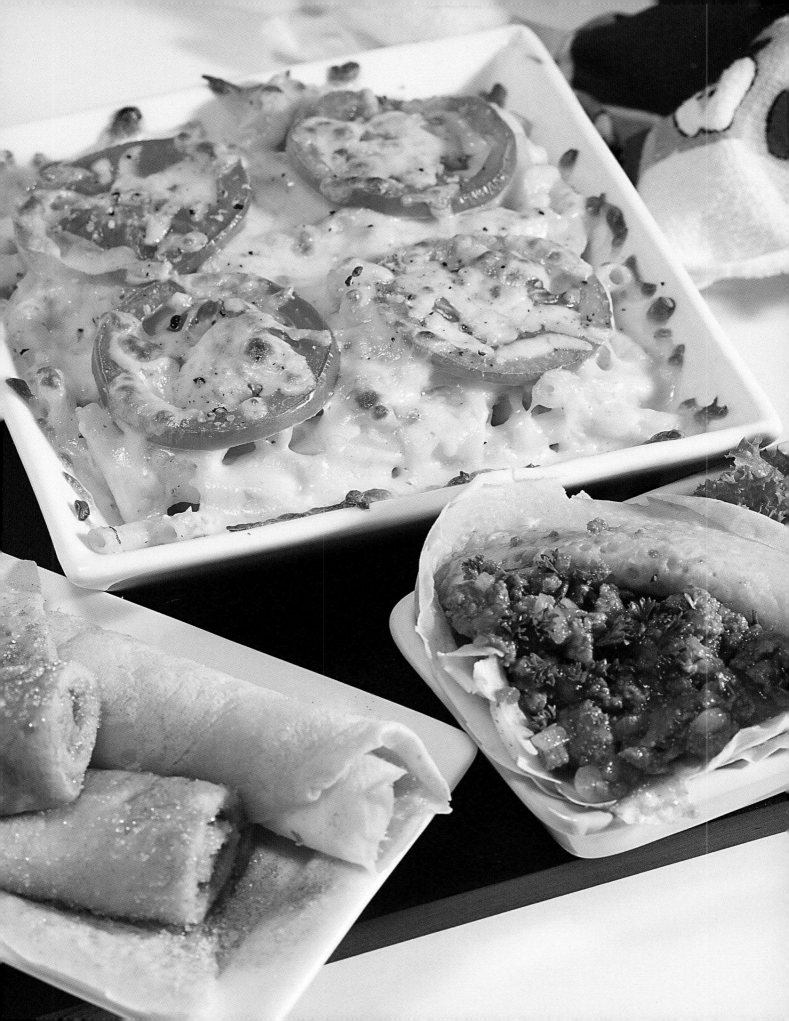

Tomato and onion quiche

Serves 6 as lunch, 12 as a tea-time treat

BASE

125 ml (½ c) high-fibre cereal*
80 ml (scant ⅓ c) warm skimmed milk*
250 ml (1 c) flour
2 ml (½ t) salt
2 ml (½ t) baking powder
1 egg
30 ml (2 T) olive or canola oil*

FILLING

3 rashers lean bacon*, flesh chopped, fat discarded
1 large onion, peeled and finely chopped
1x 410 g can baked beans in tomato sauce*
2 ml (½ t) mustard powder
2 ml (½ t) dried garlic flakes
5 ml (1 t) finely grated Parmesan
1 egg
2 egg whites
100 ml (⅖ c) skimmed milk*
150 ml (⅗ c) low-fat plain yoghurt*
salt and freshly ground pepper to taste
2 tomatoes, roughly chopped
herbs to taste (optional)
60 g low-fat mozzarella*, grated
   (2 'matchboxes' of cheese before grating)

1   First make the base. Measure out the cereal and pour the warm milk over it. Leave to stand until the cereal has softened and the milk has been absorbed.
2   Sift the flour, salt and baking powder into a mixing bowl.
3   Mash the now soft cereal and add to the flour mixture, together with the beaten egg and oil.
4   Mix carefully to a stiffish dough, using a wooden spoon.
5   Spoon the dough into a large, lightly greased quiche dish, and smooth into a thin layer with the back of a tablespoon, or using your fingertips.
6   Refrigerate for 10 minutes before adding the filling.
7   Preheat the oven to 180 °C.
8   Make the filling. Dry-fry the bacon and chopped onion until lightly browned, by adding the bacon to a clean pan, then the onion, and stirring continuously over moderate heat. There is no need to add any oil or other fat for frying as the fat from the bacon will suffice. However, if desired, you could 'fake-fry' the bacon and onion (see below).
9   While the bacon and onion are frying, place the baked beans, mustard powder, garlic and Parmesan into a liquidiser, blender or food processor, and blend until smooth, about 45 seconds.
10 Add the egg, egg whites, milk, yoghurt and seasoning, and whiz again for a few seconds to mix.
11 Place the chopped tomatoes on the chilled pastry base, and spread the onion and bacon over the tomatoes.
12 Sprinkle with herbs if desired.
13 Pour the egg and bean mixture evenly over the bacon and vegetables.
14 Sprinkle the grated mozzarella evenly over the quiche.
15 Bake for 25–30 minutes.
16 Remove from the oven, cool briefly and cut into 6 wedges to serve.

Dietician's notes

- Quiches are very high in fat. Be extra careful to use only low-fat ingredients to make sure that the fat content is as low as possible (bought quiche has 45–60 g fat per portion!).
- To reduce the fat per portion by ⅓, omit the bacon and the egg yolks, i.e. make the quiche using only the egg whites.
- Note the high fibre content due to the baked beans and the high-fibre cereal. Remember this when making your own quiches; mash a can of baked beans and add it to your filling.
- **How to fake-fry**: Pour a little good quality oil into a frying pan. Heat until the oil is hot and very liquid, but not smoking. Pick up the pan and swirl the oil around to cover the base. Pour all the oil out of the pan. Now fake-fry the food in the oil remaining in the pan.

See page 120 for Karla's creamy herb dressing, pictured right.

Nutrients per serving

Glycaemic Index 51 • Carbohydrates 37 g •
Protein 15 g • Fat 10 g • Fibre 9 g • kJ 1 279 •
Glycaemic load 18

ONE LUNCH SERVING (⅙) IS EQUIVALENT TO
1½ STARCH + 2 DAIRY/PROTEIN

ONE TEA-TIME TREAT (1/12) IS EQUIVALENT TO
1 STARCH + 1 PROTEIN

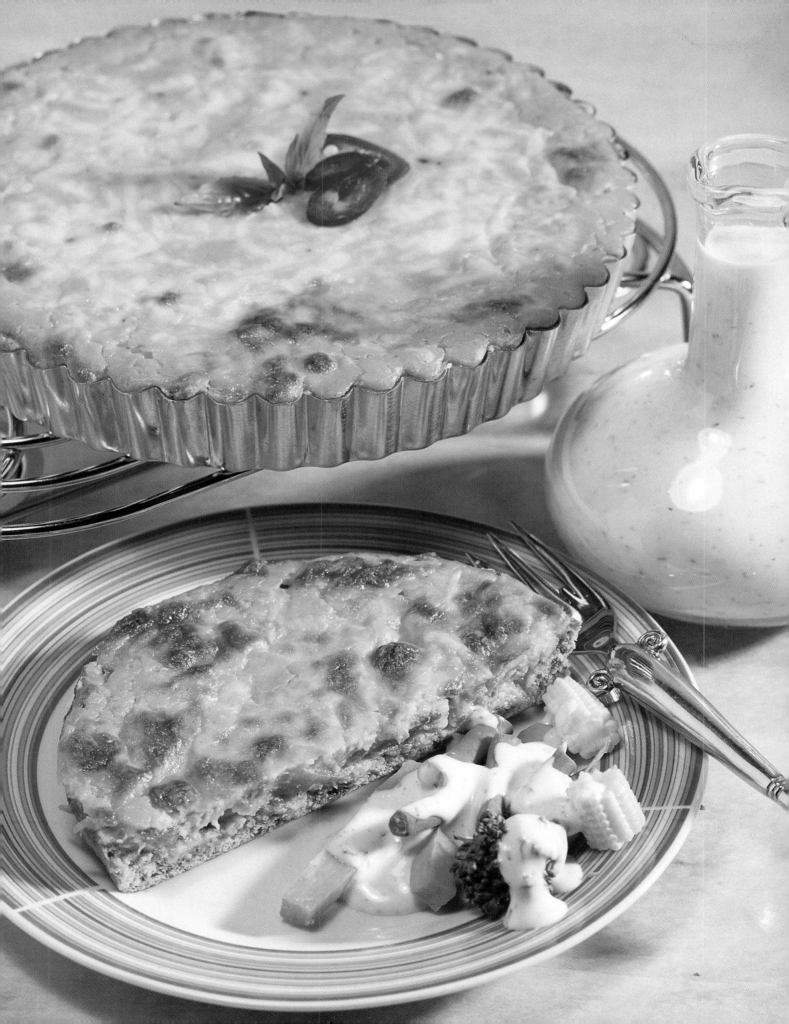

Crustless savoury tarts
Tuna and pineapple tart and Asparagus tart

Each tart serves 4

250 ml (1 c) canned or cooked butter beans*, drained
   and puréed
200 ml (⅘ c) fat-free milk*
4 eggs
10 ml (2 t) mustard powder
5 ml (1 t) salt
2 ml (½ t) freshly ground black pepper
125 ml (½ c) fresh pineapple pieces or canned
   pineapple, drained
1 x 170 g or 1 x 200 g can tuna in brine*, drained
200 g cooked asparagus or 1 x 410 g can asparagus,
   drained
120 g low-fat Cheddar cheese*, grated

This recipe makes two delicious savoury tarts without much ado.

1   Preheat the oven to 180° C and spray 2 small tart pans (23 cm in diameter) with nonstick spray.
2   Purée the drained butter beans with 100 ml (⅖ c) of the milk.
3   Pour into a bowl and add the rest of the milk, the eggs, mustard powder, salt and pepper, and stir to mix.
4   Halve the egg and milk mixture (pour half into another bowl), then add the pineapple and tuna to 1 half. Mix gently.
5   Pour the tuna and pineapple filling into 1 tart dish.
6   Pour enough of the remaining egg and milk mixture into the second tart dish to be about 2 mm deep, then spread the asparagus pieces evenly over the second tart dish and pour over the remaining milk and egg mix.
7   Sprinkle the grated cheese evenly over the 2 tarts.
8   Place both tarts carefully into the oven and bake for 35 minutes, or until set.
9   Leave to cool slightly and serve with a tossed salad and low-oil dressing, and 1 slice of low GI Health bread (page 96), if desired.

If you do not like pineapple with the tuna, leave it out, or use onion instead.
Any leftover cooked vegetables can be used in place of the asparagus.
Should you only eat 1 of the tarts, the other can be frozen successfully.

Dietician's notes

- We have used puréed butter beans instead of flour to thicken and set these savoury tarts, as flour has a very high GI.
- Because of the soluble fibre in the beans, the entire dish has a lower GI. Using beans in this way is quick and easy to do and much healthier.
- Remember to use the lower fat cheese, as this is the main source of fat in these tart recipes.
- Note the extremely low Glycaemic load (GL) of both tarts. This means that a lunch planned with these tarts as the main component will have a very small impact on blood glucose levels.
- Should you prefer not to eat bread with these tarts, you can choose a lower GI starch-containing snack, e.g. Nina's chocolate date squares (page 114) or a muffin of your choice (pages 26–28) instead of a fruit for the next snack.

See page 122 for the Party fruit punch recipe, pictured opposite.

Nutrients per serving
Tuna and pineapple tart
Glycaemic Index 41 • Carbohydrates 9 g •
Protein 17 g • Fat 7 g • Fibre 3 g • kJ 702 •
Glycaemic load 4

ONE SERVING TUNA AND PINEAPPLE TART IS
EQUIVALENT TO ½ STARCH + 2 PROTEIN

Nutrients per serving
Asparagus tart
Glycaemic Index <40 • Carbohydrates 8 g •
Protein 11 g • Fat 6 g • Fibre 3 g • kJ 567 •
Glycaemic load 2

ONE SERVING ASPARAGUS TART IS EQUIVALENT TO
½ STARCH +1½ PROTEIN + VEGETABLE

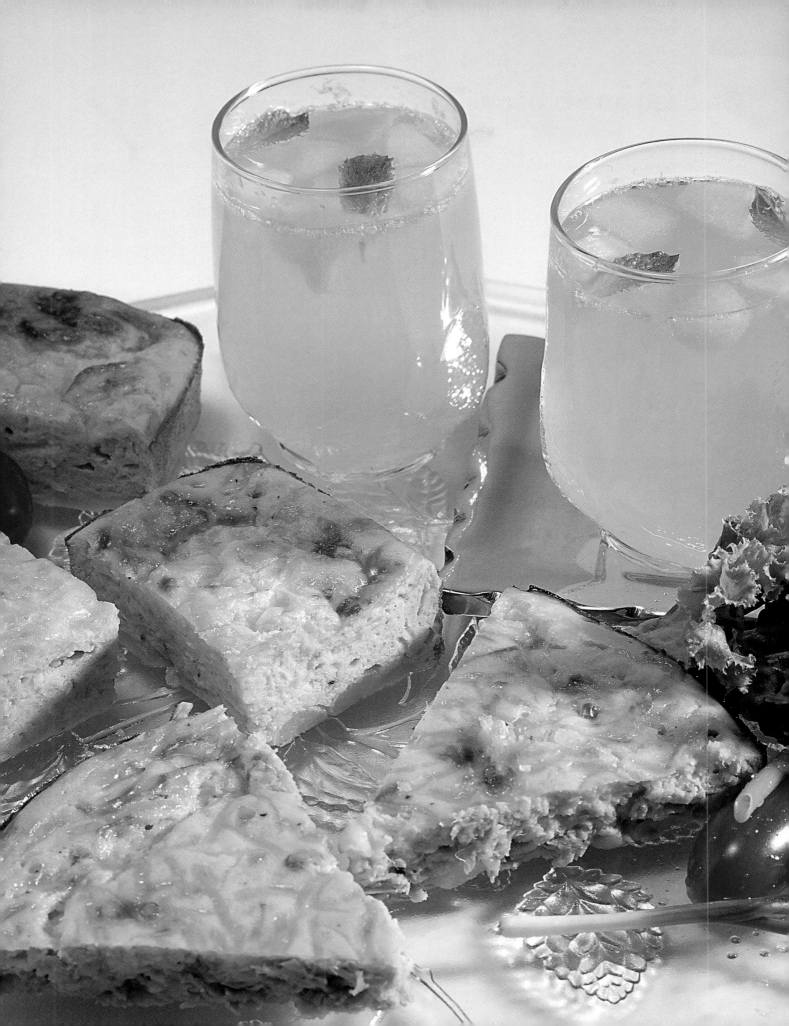

Chicken and broccoli casserole

Serves 4

1 large head broccoli or 500 g frozen broccoli
400 g cooked chicken breasts, shredded (500 ml [2 c])
375 ml (1½ c) chicken stock, reserved from cooking
   the chicken
60 ml (4 T) flour
1 ml (¼ t) salt
2 ml (½ t) freshly ground black pepper
1 ml (¼ t) grated nutmeg
60 g mozzarella*, grated (2 'matchboxes' of cheese
   before grating)
65 ml (¼ c) fat-free plain yoghurt*
1 ml (¼ t) cayenne pepper
5 ml (1 t) Worcester sauce

1 If you are using fresh broccoli, wash the broccoli and cut into bite-sized florets (makes about 1.25 litres [5 cups] florets). Place the florets in a sieve and gradually pour a whole kettleful of boiling water over the florets to blanch them, letting the hot water run down into the sink.
2 Layer the blanched broccoli and the chicken in a greased casserole dish.
3 Preheat the oven to 200 °C.
4 Make the sauce. Bring the stock to the boil in a saucepan.
5 Mix the flour with 50 ml (⅕ c) water to make a smooth paste.
6 Add a little boiling stock to the flour and water paste, stirring continuously.
7 Gradually add the resulting paste to the rest of the boiling stock, stirring well with a whisk to make a smooth sauce. Add the salt, black pepper and grated nutmeg. Boil over moderate heat until thick and smooth.
8 Remove from the stove; stir in half the cheese and all the yoghurt, the cayenne pepper and the Worcester sauce.
9 Pour the sauce over broccoli and chicken and sprinkle with remaining cheese.
10 Bake for 20 minutes, or until heated through and the topping is bubbly.
11 Cook 185 ml (¾ c) lower GI rice* and serve with the casserole.

Variation: Instead of rice, serve with 250 ml (1 c) mashed potatoes mixed with 250 ml (1 c) canned lentil or pea dhal. Season with salt, black pepper and nutmeg.

Dietician's notes

- The analysis alongside is for the chicken, broccoli and the low GI starch.
- Note that the recipe calls for 1.25 litres (5 c) of broccoli and only 500 ml (2 c) of chicken. In SA we generally eat too much protein and too few vegetables. This recipe has the correct ratio.

Nutrients per serving
(Casserole with rice)
Glycaemic Index 55 • Carbohydrates 38 g •
Protein 40 g • Fat 8 g • Fibre 4 g • kJ 1 680 •
Glycaemic load 21

ONE SERVING OF CHICKEN CASSEROLE AND RICE
(OR MASH) IS EQUIVALENT TO 2 STARCH + 4 LEAN
PROTEIN/DAIRY + VEGETABLES

Unbelievable chicken

Serves 4

1–2 pieces chicken per person, e.g. 1 breast or
   1 drumstick plus 1 thigh per person
60 ml (4 T) low-fat mayonnaise*
60 ml (4 T) chutney, preferably 'lite'
15 g (⅓ packet) onion soup powder or 15 ml (1 T) onion
   soup powder and 15 ml (1 T) oat bran
boiling water

1 Preheat the oven to 220 °C.
2 Remove all fat and skin from the chicken, and place in an ovenproof dish.
3 Mix the mayonnaise, chutney and soup powder in a cup or mug. Add enough boiling water to fill the cup or mug, and mix well. Pour over the chicken.
4 Cover the dish and bake the chicken for 30 minutes.
5 Remove the lid and bake until browned, turning often. Add water if necessary.
6 Serve with fresh sweetcorn (halved corn on the cob) and vegetables, e.g. Stuffed butternut (page 72) and tomato salad.

Variation: Place sliced mushrooms, chopped onion or other vegetables in the base of the dish before adding the chicken and sauce.

Dietician's notes

- This is the favourite chicken dish of Liesbet's family, and we're sure that your family will also want to eat it again and again!
- Serving the chicken with sweetcorn offers an interesting, low GI alternative starch to rice and potatoes, which one is more inclined to use.
- Remember that the packet soup mix is high in sodium, which should be eaten in moderation by those suffering from high blood pressure. Make sure you have no other high sodium foods on the same day as eating this dish.

Nutrients per portion
(Chicken and sweetcorn)
Glycaemic index 53 • Carbohydrates 26 g •
Protein 31 g • Fat 7 g • Fibre 3 g • kJ 1 226 •
Glycaemic load 14

ONE SERVING OF CHICKEN AND SWEETCORN IS
EQUIVALENT TO 3 LEAN PROTEIN + 1½ STARCH

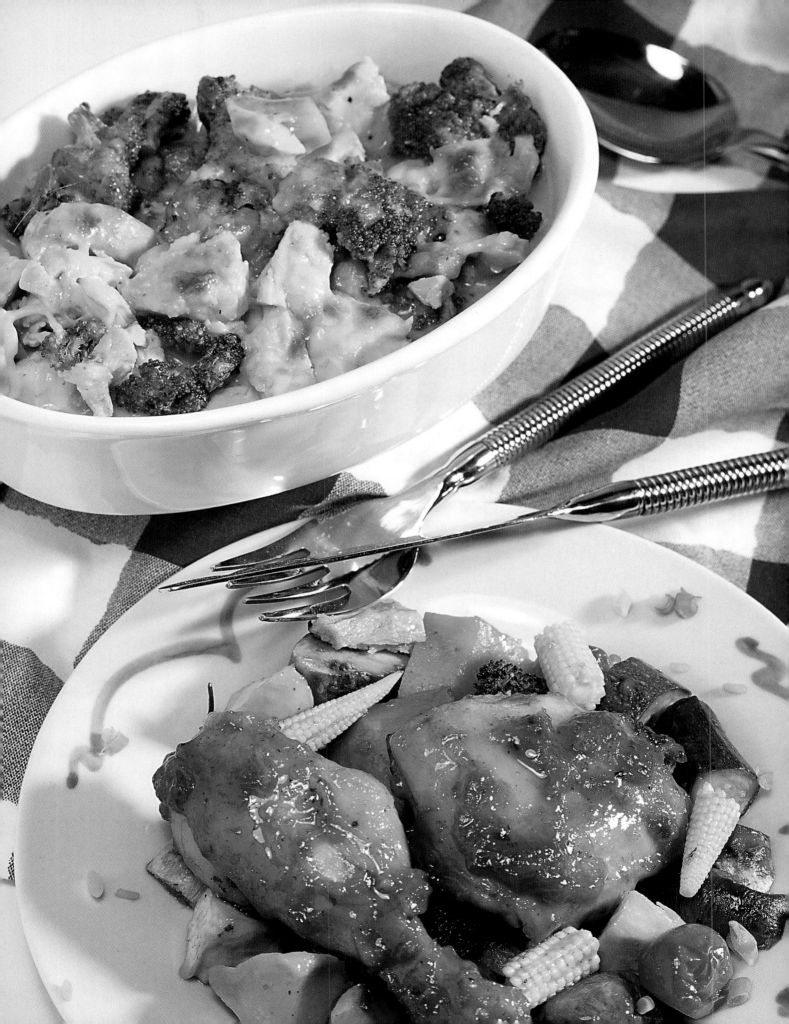

Mango chicken

Serves 4

5 ml (1 t) olive or canola oil*

4 chicken breast fillets, cubed (500 g)

1 bunch spring onions, sliced or 1 onion, peeled and
    chopped

2 cloves garlic, crushed or 5 ml (1 t) dried garlic flakes

15–30 ml (1–2 T) medium-strength curry powder

250 ml (1 c) chicken stock or ½ stock cube or 10 ml
    (2 t) stock powder dissolved in 250 ml (1 c) boiling
    water

1 fresh mango (250 g), peeled and chopped
    or 1 x 410 g can mangoes, drained and chopped

freshly ground pepper to taste

60 ml (4 T) low-fat or fat-free plain yoghurt*

Nutrients per serving
(Chicken and barley)
Glycaemic Index <40 • Carbohydrates 38 g •
Protein 32 g • Fat 6 g • Fibre 6 g • kJ 1 474 •
Glycaemic load 11

ONE SERVING OF CHICKEN AND BARLEY IS EQUIVALENT
TO 4 LEAN PROTEIN + 1½ STARCH + ½ FRUIT

1 Heat the oil in a large frying pan.
2 Add the chicken cubes and fry over high heat, turning occasionally, until browned
   on all sides.
3 Remove from the pan and set aside.
4 Add the spring onions or onion, garlic and curry powder. Stir-fry for 1 minute.
5 Add the chicken stock and mango and season to taste with salt and freshly
   ground black pepper.
6 Simmer for 5 minutes, return the chicken to the pan and cook until heated.
7 Stir in the yoghurt and remove from the heat. Do not boil or the yoghurt will
   curdle.
8 Serve hot with cooked barley, lower GI rice or low GI fettuccine (185 ml [¾ c]
   uncooked to serve 4). Add a gem squash per person and a mixed salad for the
   perfect meal.

This is a deliciously different curried chicken, and can be served either hot or cold.

Dietician's notes

- The higher GI mango is compensated for by the low GI starch, vegetables and
  the yoghurt.
- We have used low-fat yoghurt in place of the traditional full-fat cream, to retain
  the creamy texture of the dish, but lower the fat content. Alternatively, one could
  use pouring cream that is also lower in fat, but then use half the quantity.

Mustard chicken

Serves 4

15 ml (1 T) sugar

5 ml (1 t) mustard powder

15 ml (1 T) cake flour

15 ml (1 T) canola oil

15 ml (1 T) vinegar

50 ml (⅕ c) lower fat mayonnaise*

200 ml (⅘ c) boiling water

500 g chicken breast fillets, cubed or 1 chicken
    drumstick and 1 chicken thigh, skinned, per person

Nutrients per serving
(Chicken and rice)
Glycaemic Index 55 • Carbohydrates 26 g •
Protein 30 g • Fat 6 g • Fibre 2 g • kJ 1 238 •
Glycaemic load 15

ONE SERVING OF CHICKEN AND RICE IS EQUIVALENT TO
3 LEAN PROTEIN + 1½ STARCH

1 Preheat the oven to 200 °C.
2 Mix the sugar, mustard powder and cake flour.
3 Add the oil and vinegar and stir well.
4 Add the mayonnaise and water and mix well, using a whisk, to make a sauce.
5 Place the chicken pieces in a medium casserole dish and pour the sauce over.
   Bake, covered, for 30 minutes.
6 Remove the covering and turn the chicken pieces. Bake, uncovered, for 30 minutes, or until the chicken pieces have browned and the sauce has thickened.
7 Boil 185 ml (¾ c) brown rice* (enough to serve 4).
8 Serve the chicken and rice with a vegetable, e.g. one of the vegetable duos (page
   76), and beetroot salad.

*This is another tasty chicken dish, which has such a lovely sauce that you won't even
miss the chicken skin!*

Dietician's notes

- Basmati rice or any other lower GI rice can be used instead of brown rice, but
  the fibre content of the meal will then be lower, and the kilojoule count a little
  higher.
- Again, this recipe shows how combining a small quantity of high GI ingredients
  (flour and sugar) with lower GI ingredients (brown rice and vegetables) results in
  a low GI meal.

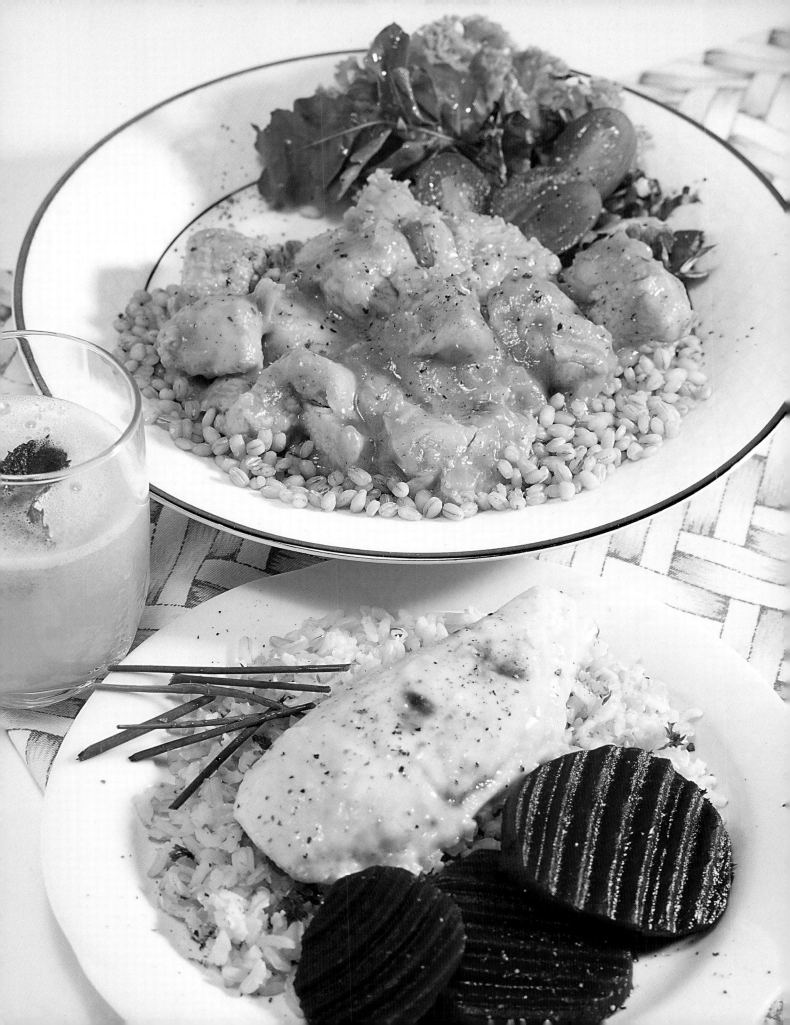

Peachy chicken casserole

Serves 6

100 ml (⅖ c) uncooked split lentils*
125 ml (½ c) hot water
6 chicken breasts, skinned
5 ml (1 t) paprika
freshly ground black pepper to taste
5 ml (1 t) olive or canola oil*
1 onion, peeled and chopped
250 g mushrooms, sliced
1 x 62 g packet creamy mushroom soup
250 ml (1 c) peach or peach and orange juice*
125 ml (½ c) water

Nutrients per serving
(Chicken and wheat rice)
Glycaemic Index 48 • Carbohydrates 41 g •
Protein 35 g • Fat 9 g • Fibre 7 g • kJ 1 502 •
Glycaemic load 20

ONE SERVING OF CHICKEN AND WHEAT RICE IS
EQUIVALENT TO
3 LEAN PROTEIN + 2 STARCH + 1 VEGETABLE/FRUIT

1 Layer the lentils evenly in the base of a casserole dish. Carefully pour the hot water over the lentils. Leave to soak for 10 minutes. Preheat the oven to 180 °C.
2 Place the skinned chicken breasts in a single layer on top of the lentils and water, and dust the chicken breasts lightly with paprika and pepper.
3 Pour the oil into a saucepan; heat gently and then fry the onion until transparent. Add the mushrooms, and fry until most of the liquid has evaporated.
4 Mix together the soup powder, peach juice and water until smooth, and pour over the mushrooms and onions. Stir over moderate heat until the sauce thickens.
5 Pour over the chicken pieces, cover and bake for 30 minutes, then stir to mix the lentils into the sauce.
6 Add a little water if the sauce is too thick. Return to the oven and bake for a further 30 minutes; remove the lid or covering and bake for another 30 minutes, or until the chicken has browned.
7 Serve with boiled wheat rice* (375 ml [1½ c] uncooked to serve 6), mixed with a little chopped mint.
8 Add a large mixed salad or 2 cooked vegetables and you will have a balanced, low GI, low-fat meal, fit for a king.

Dietician's notes

- Take note of the small meat portion. In spite of this, the fat count is still 9 g.
- Note that we have used a very high GI, convenient, powdered soup mix. By combining it with the low GI split lentils, fruit juice, vegetables, wheat rice and salad, the GI of the whole meal is effectively lowered.

Tandoori chicken

Serves 4

1–2 chicken thighs or 1 chicken breast per person
vegetables, e.g. chunks of red or green sweet peppers
  or sundried tomatoes, soaked in water
MARINADE
1 onion, peeled and grated
250 ml (1 c) low-fat or fat-free plain yoghurt*
5 ml (1 t) turmeric
5 ml (1 t) paprika
5 ml (1 t) masala
2 ml (½ t) ground coriander
2 ml (½ t) ground ginger
10 ml (2 t) lemon juice
1 clove garlic, chopped or 5 ml (1 t) dried garlic flakes
1 ml (¼ t) salt
5 ml (1 t) sugar

Nutrients per serving (Chicken and rice)
Glycaemic Index 42 • Carbohydrates 37 g •
Protein 33 g • Fat 5 g • Fibre 1 g • kJ 1 353 •
Glycaemic load 15

ONE SERVING OF CHICKEN AND RICE IS EQUIVALENT TO
3 LEAN PROTEIN + 2 STARCH

1 Soak 4 bamboo skewers in water for several hours. This will prevent them from burning when the kebabs are grilled in the oven or on the braai.
2 Remove all skin and visible fat from the chicken pieces.
3 Prick the chicken meat well all over, cut into cubes and place in a shallow dish.
4 Combine all the marinade ingredients in a jug and pour over the chicken.
5 Store, covered with plastic wrap or a lid, in the refrigerator for 3 hours or over-night, stirring occasionally.
6 Drain the chicken and reserve the marinade.
7 Thread the chicken pieces onto the skewers, alternating with the vegetables, and place in a roasting pan.
8 Grill under a hot grill until tender and well-browned or braai out of doors, turning every 2–3 minutes and basting occasionally with the reserved marinade.
9 Serve with rice or barley (for 4 servings, cook 185 ml [¾ c] uncooked rice or barley) and vegetables or green banana, cucumber and yoghurt salad, as well as tomato salad or sambals. (The GI will be lower if barley is used.)

Variation: The thighs or breasts can be marinated whole in the tandoori mixture. Roast in the oven at 180 °C for 1 hour, turning often and basting occasionally.

Dietician's note

- The analysis alongside is for chicken breasts. If thighs are used the fat content will be higher, but still below 10 g per serving.

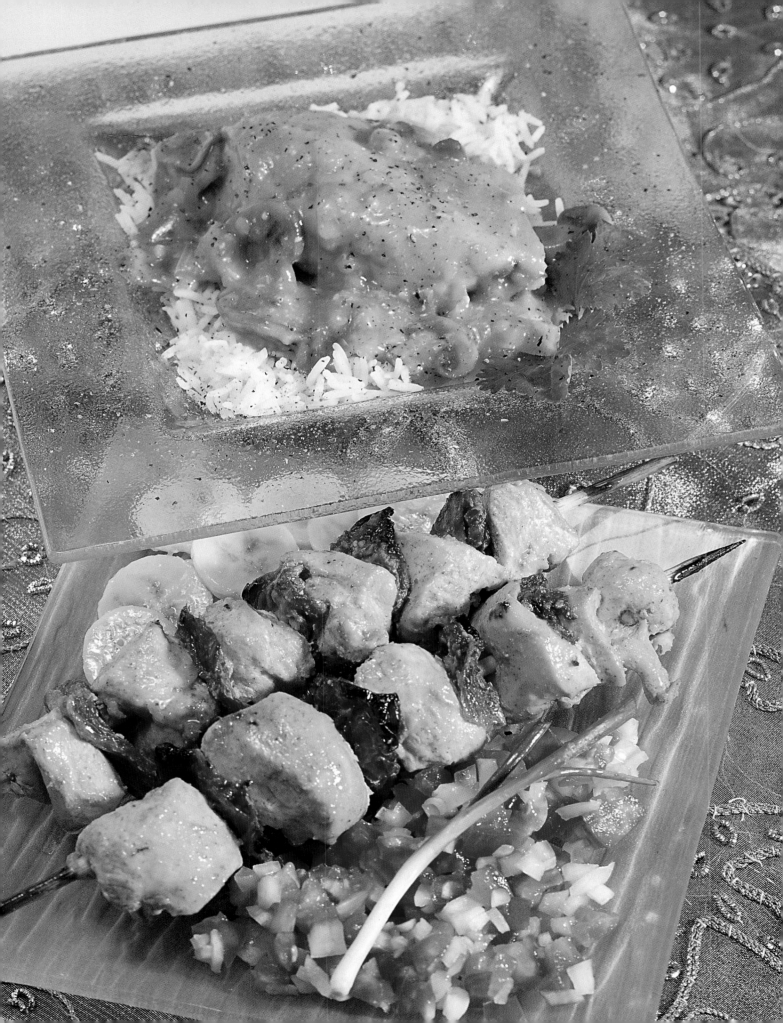

Satay chicken (kebabs)

Serves 4

500 g chicken breasts, skinned
vegetables e.g. onion slices, whole button
    mushrooms, etc
MARINADE
1 clove garlic, crushed
65 ml (¼ c) soy sauce
65 ml (¼ c) lemon juice
½ small onion, peeled and grated

1 Cut skinned chicken into cubes large enough not to tear apart on a skewer, and place in a shallow dish.
2 In a glass bowl, mix the garlic, soy sauce, lemon juice and onion; microwave the marinade on high for 1–2 minutes to cook the onion.
3 Pour over the chicken kebabs and marinate for at least 1 hour, but preferably overnight.
4 Thread the chicken onto skewers, alternating with vegetables of your choice.
5 Braai or grill the kebabs, turning every 2–3 minutes, until just done. Be careful not to overcook them as they will dry out.
6 Serve with 45 ml (3T) satay (peanut) sauce per kebab, lower GI rice* (185 ml [¾ c] uncooked rice to serve 4) and a salad or cooked vegetables e.g. Cabbage stir-fry (page 68).

Soak skewers in water for 1 hour to prevent burning.

Nutrients per marinated kebab
(no satay sauce)
Carbohydrates 2 g • Protein 28 g • Fat 4 g • Fibre negl. • kJ 673

ONE MARINATED KEBAB WITHOUT SAUCE IS EQUIVALENT TO 3 LEAN PROTEIN

Nutrients per kebab with rice
(no satay sauce)
Glycaemic index 48 • Carbohydrates 30 g • Protein 31 g • Fat 4 g • Fibre 1 g • kJ 1 212 • Glycaemic load 14

ONE KEBAB WITH RICE (NO SAUCE) IS EQUIVALENT TO 2 STARCH + 3 LEAN PROTEIN

Peanut sauce (Satay sauce)

Serves 8 Makes 350 ml

15 ml (1 T) water
½ small onion, peeled and finely grated
1 clove garlic
2 ml (½ t) chilli
60 ml (4 T) peanut butter
15 ml (1 T) soy sauce
15–30 ml (1–2 T) lime or lemon juice
250 ml (1 c) water, or a 50:50 mixture of apple juice*
    and water (for a sweeter sauce)

1 Bring the water, onion and garlic to the boil in a small saucepan, and cook gently.
2 Add the chilli and cook for another 3 minutes.
3 Add the peanut butter, 15 ml (1 T) at a time, stirring well after each addition, to make a smooth sauce.
4 Add the soy sauce, lime or lemon juice and half the water or water and apple juice mixture, and mix well. Add the rest of the water or water and apple juice mixture and stir well.
5 Bring to the boil, stirring constantly.
6 Reduce the heat and simmer the sauce for 2 minutes.
7 Spoon 45 ml (3 T) Satay sauce over each kebab (refrigerate or freeze the rest of the sauce for another meal).

This sauce keeps well in the fridge for one week.

Dietician's notes
- Satay peanut sauce is usually too high in fat, but if you reduce the quantity of peanut butter and use water or water and apple juice to dilute it as we did, it is quite acceptable.
- Peanuts contain mainly monounsaturated fats, which are beneficial fats.

Nutrients per kebab with Satay sauce and rice
Glycaemic index 45 • Carbohydrates 32 g • Protein 33 g • Fat 9 g • Fibre 1 g • kJ 1 477 • Glycaemic load 14

ONE KEBAB WITH SAUCE AND RICE IS EQUIVALENT TO 2 STARCH + 3 LEAN PROTEIN + 1 FAT

Nutrients per 45 ml (3 T) Satay sauce
Carbohydrates 2 g • Protein 3 g • Fat 5 g • Fibre negl. • kJ 265
ONE SERVING OF SATAY SAUCE IS EQUIVALENT TO 1 FAT

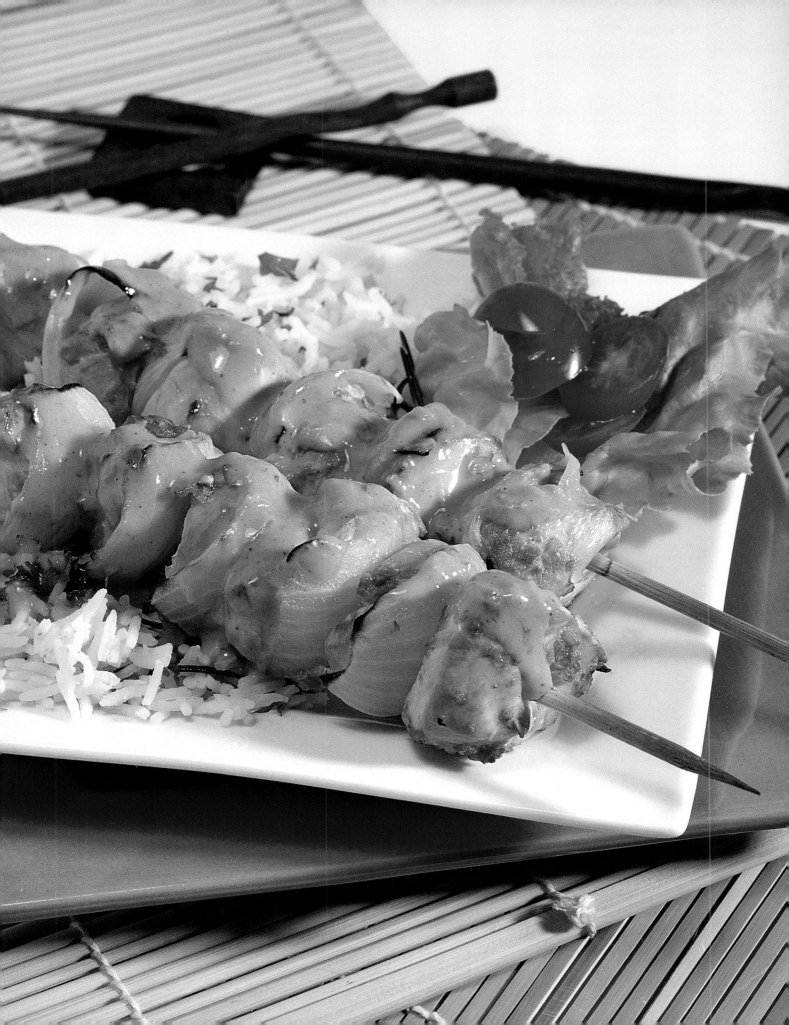

Thai chicken and vegetable curry

Serves 4

185 ml (¾ c) uncooked basmati rice
5 ml (1 t) salt
500 ml (2 c) water
4 chicken breast fillets, cut into strips
10 ml (2 t) Thai red curry paste
5 ml (1 t) canola, olive or macadamia oil*
1 large clove garlic, crushed
1 litre (4 c) chopped cabbage (400 g)
500 ml (2 c) broccoli, cut into small florets (200 g)
100 ml (¼ x 400 ml can) 'lite' coconut milk*
100 ml (⅖ c) skimmed milk*
15 ml (1 T) tomato sauce
15 ml (1 T) soy sauce or fish sauce
15 ml (1 T) lemon or lime juice
15 ml (1 T) soft brown sugar
10–15 ml (2–3 t) finely chopped fresh basil
10 ml (2 t) gravy powder
45 ml (3 T) water

1 Bring the rice, salt and 500 ml (2 c) water to the boil in a covered saucepan.
2 Turn the heat right down and simmer for 30 minutes, or until all the liquid has been absorbed by the rice. Leave the lid slightly askew on the saucepan, otherwise the rice will boil over.
3 While the rice is cooking, coat the chicken pieces on both sides with the curry paste, using your fingers.
4 Heat the oil in a large wok or frying pan until quite hot, but not smoking.
5 Add the garlic and chicken and stir-fry until the chicken browns slightly.
6 Add the cabbage and broccoli and stir-fry until the cabbage browns slightly.
7 Add the coconut milk, milk and tomato sauce and stir. Cover, bring to the boil and simmer for 5–10 minutes, or until the broccoli is tender but not limp.
8 Add the soy sauce or fish sauce, lemon or lime juice, sugar and basil.
9 Stir to combine and cook until heated through.
10 Mix the gravy powder with 45 ml (3 T) water to make a smooth paste. Add to the curry to thicken it slightly.
11 Serve on the cooked basmati rice.

This is a delicious dish, if you have all the Thai ingredients on hand.

The typical Thai flavour is easily achieved by using Thai curry paste, fish sauce, brown sugar and basil together with the coconut milk. Most supermarkets now stock the Thai red curry paste, the fish sauce, 'lite' coconut milk and fresh, dried or bottled basil.

For a vegetarian curry, leave out the chicken and replace with 1 x 410 g can chickpeas, drained, and an extra 250 ml (1 c) vegetables.

Dietician's notes

* Any vegetables can be used in this recipe: green beans, cabbage, broccoli, celery, cauliflower, carrots, mushrooms, sugar-snap peas, courgettes, etc, as long as you use a total of 1.5 litres (6 c) uncooked chopped vegetables.
* Coconut milk is rather high in saturated fat and not really suitable for good health, but it is an essential ingredient in Thai cooking. For this reason, we have compromised by using half skimmed milk and half 'lite' coconut milk, which is lower in fat (there is only 1 g of saturated fat per portion when you use 'lite' coconut milk).
* Should you prefer not to use coconut milk, or if you cannot find it, you can use 200 ml (⅘ c) lower fat evaporated milk with 100 ml (⅖ c) water and 8 drops of coconut essence.
* Although gravy powder has a very high GI, it is safe to use in this recipe as all the other low GI ingredients cancel out the effect of the high GI gravy powder.
* Remember that this is a whole meal and therefore the fat content of 10 g per portion and a GL of 20 is quite acceptable.
* Note that the GL of a portion of most cooked starches (baby potato, sweet potato, rice or pasta) varies from 10–15 per portion. This means that the starch makes the greatest contribution to the GL of a meal.

Nutrients per serving
(Thai curry and rice)
Glycaemic Index 52 • Carbohydrates 39 g •
Protein 32 g • Fat 10 g • Fibre 4 g • kJ 1 625 •
Glycaemic load 20

ONE SERVING OF THAI CURRY AND RICE IS EQUIVALENT
TO 2 STARCH + 3 PROTEIN/DAIRY + VEGETABLES

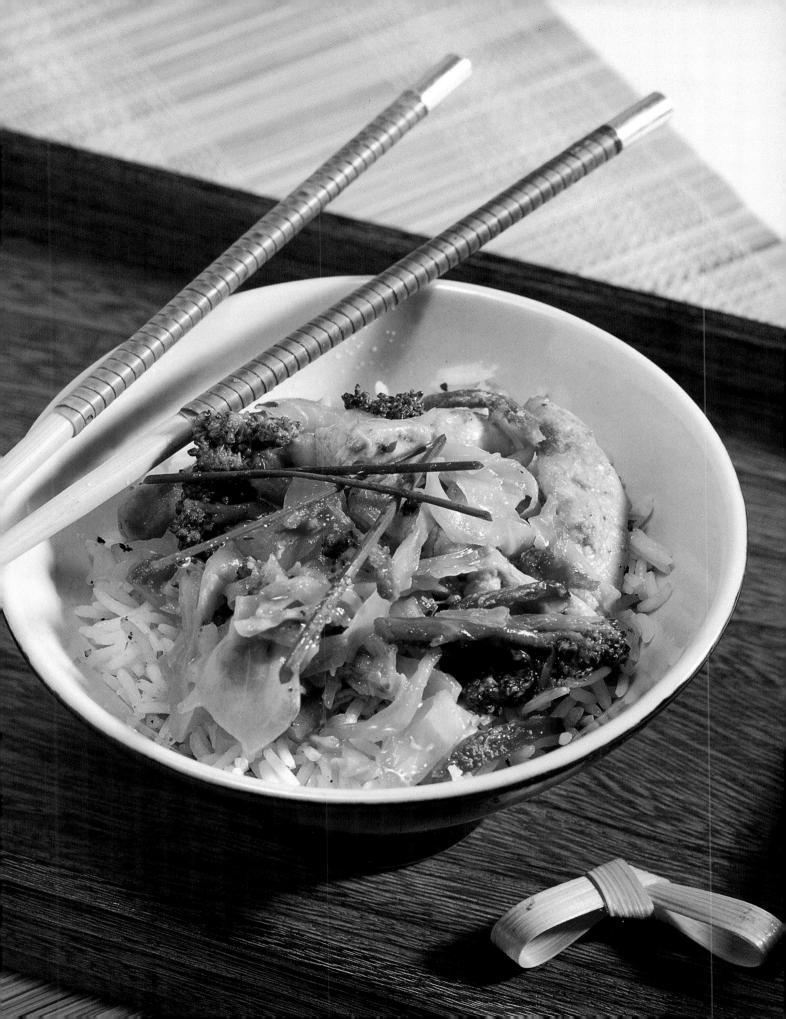

Fish bobotie

Serves 4

400 g frozen hake fillets or other firm-fleshed white
  fish, slightly defrosted and skin removed
250 ml (1 c) fat-free or skimmed milk*
5 ml (1 t) olive or canola oil
1 large onion, peeled and chopped
1 clove garlic, chopped or 2 ml (½ t) garlic flakes
30 ml (2 T) chutney ('lite', if desired)
10 ml (2 t) curry powder
5 ml (1 t) masala
5 ml (1 t) turmeric
30 g (80 ml or scant ⅓ c) lower GI oats*
60 ml (4 T) sultanas
25 ml (5 t) freshly squeezed lemon juice
2 ml (½ t) salt and freshly ground pepper to taste
1 egg
fresh lemon leaves or dried bay leaves

1   Preheat the oven to 180 °C.
2   Poach the fish in 125 ml (½ c) of the milk for 10–15 minutes, or until done.
3   In the meantime, heat the oil in a frying pan.
4   Add the onion and garlic, and fry until the onion is transparent.
5   Add the chutney, curry powder, masala, turmeric and oats, and fry lightly.
6   Add the onion mixture, sultanas, lemon juice, and salt and pepper to the cooked fish and milk, and mix thoroughly; spoon into a greased, ovenproof dish.
7   Add the egg to the remainder of the milk and beat together until well combined. Add half to the fish mixture, and mix it in lightly.
8   Pour the remaining milk and egg mixture over the fish, press the lemon leaves or bay leaves into the fish bobotie, and bake the bobotie, in the centre of the oven for 20 minutes, or until the egg and milk mixture has set.
9   Serve hot with lower GI rice (e.g. Tastic or basmati rice), barley or pearled wheat (boil about 190 ml [¾ c] to serve 4), and green banana, tomato and onion, and Cucumber salad (page 34).

Chopped dried apricots (6–8) may be used instead of the sultanas.
  Bobotie is a traditional Malayan dish: onion, garlic, curry powder, masala, turmeric and chutney give this dish its typical flavour.

Dietician's notes

- This is a tasty, low-fat alternative to regular bobotie.
- The nutritional analysis is for the bobotie with rice. The GI and GL would be lower if the bobotie were eaten with pearled barley, or 'stampkoring'.
- Women may want to eat only 1 portion of starch, so dish up a little more rice or other starch for the men.

Nutrients per serving
(Bobotie and rice)
Glycaemic Index 48 • Carbohydrates 49 g •
Protein 25 g • Fat 5 g • Fibre 3 g • kJ 1 431 •
Glycaemic load 24

ONE SERVING OF BOBOTIE AND RICE IS EQUIVALENT TO
3 LEAN PROTEIN + 2 STARCH + 1 VEGETABLE

Hake mornay

Serves 4

400 g (1 packet) hake or kabeljou fillets, skin removed
5 ml (1 t) chicken stock powder
250 ml (1 c) skimmed milk*
2 eggs
30 g lower fat cheese*, grated
l5 ml (1 T) low-fat margarine*, melted

1   Preheat the oven to 180 °C.
2   Place the fish in a lightly greased ovenproof dish.
3   Sprinkle the chicken stock powder over the fish.
4   Beat the milk and eggs together and pour over the fish.
5   Sprinkle the cheese on top and pour over the melted margarine.
6   Bake in the oven until the egg mixture has set, about 30 minutes.
7   Serve with a low GI starch e.g. 3 – 5 baby potatoes (with skin) per person and 2–3 vegetables (e.g. green peas, gem squash, sautéed mushrooms, etc.) or salads.

Hake mornay is usually made with a rich cheese sauce. This sauce is a fresh and healthier alternative.

Dietician's note

- The GI and GL have been calculated with the baby potatoes included. Without potatoes, the dish would not really have a GI, as the GI and GL refer only to carbohydrate-rich foods.

Nutrients per serving
(Fish with the starch)
Glycaemic Index 55 • Carbohydrates 27 g •
Protein 27 g • Fat 7 g • Fibre 2 g • kJ 1 203 •
Glycaemic load 15

ONE SERVING OF FISH AND BABY POTATOES IS
EQUIVALENT TO 3 LEAN PROTEIN + 1½ STARCH

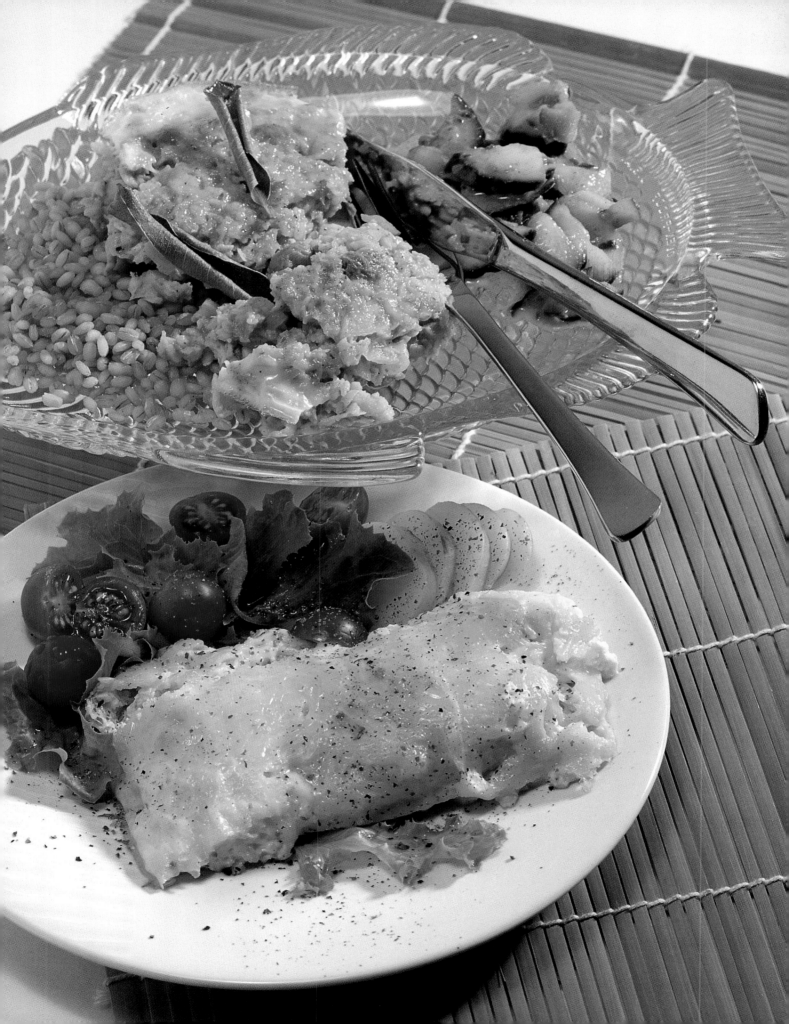

Fish pie

Serves 4

CRUST

5–7 (200 g) baby potatoes with skin

1 x 225 g can baked beans in tomato sauce*, drained

1 egg white, whisked

5 ml (1 t) baking powder

60 ml (4 T) oat bran*

FILLING

5 ml (1 t) oil

1 large onion, peeled and finely chopped

1 x 410 g can pilchards in tomato sauce

60 ml (4 T) low-fat mayonnaise*

60 ml (4 T) finely chopped fresh parsley or 2 ml (½ t)
    dried herbs of your choice

15 ml (1 T) vinegar or lemon juice

1 egg, beaten

2 ml (½ t) dried garlic flakes or 1 clove garlic

30 g (1 'matchbox') low-fat cheese*, grated

Nutrients per serving

Glycaemic Index 48 • Carbohydrates 30 g •
Protein 27 g • Fat 12 g • Fibre 7 g • kJ 1 373 •
Glycaemic load 15

ONE SERVING OF FISH PIE IS EQUIVALENT TO
1½ STARCH + 3 PROTEIN

1 Preheat the oven to 180 °C.

2 Chop the unpeeled baby potatoes into cubes and boil in lightly salted water (or microwave) until soft. Drain and place in a liquidiser or blender.

3 Add the drained baked beans and the egg white, and purée for 1–2 minutes. Add the baking powder and oat bran and mix well.

4 Spray a shallow 1.5 litre ovenproof dish with nonstick spray.

5 Spread the potato mixture on the base and sides of the dish and set aside.

6 Heat the oil in a frying pan and fry the chopped onion until transparent.

7 Drain the pilchards, keeping the tomato sauce for garnishing, and gently mash with a fork. Mix together the pilchards, mayonnaise, fried onion, parsley or dried herbs, vinegar or lemon juice, egg and garlic.

8 Spoon the mixture into the potato crust.

9 Drizzle the tomato sauce from the baked beans and the pilchards over the filling and spread it out evenly. Sprinkle the grated cheese on top.

10 Bake the pie for 20–30 minutes on the middle shelf of the oven.

11 Serve hot or cold with vegetables or salad (e.g. Green bean relish, page 36). No starch is required, as it is already included in the crust of this pie.

Dietician's notes

• This is a good example of how low GI beans can be used to lower the GI of higher GI potatoes, without losing too much on taste.

• The soft bones of the pilchards are a good source of calcium; 100 g of pilchards contain as much calcium as a glass of milk!

• Pilchards are a good source of omega 3 essential fatty acids, which are especially good for those suffering from allergies, asthma, ADHD and arthritis.

• The fat content is at the higher end of the recommended range per meal, but since most of this fat comes from omega-3 fats, this is quite acceptable.

Hake with apricot sauce

Serves 4

5 ml (1 t) oil

1 small onion, peeled and finely chopped

1 clove garlic, chopped or 2 ml (½ t) dried garlic flakes

1 ml (¼ t) curry powder

1 ml (¼ t) ground cinnamon

1 ml (¼ t) ground ginger

30 ml (2 T) lower GI oats*

250 ml (1 c) apricot or other lower GI juice*

500 g hake fillets, frozen

pinch of salt

Nutrients per serving
(Fish and pearled wheat)

Glycaemic Index 45 • Carbohydrates 32 g •
Protein 27 g • Fat 3 g • Fibre 8 g • kJ 1 222 •
Glycaemic load 15

ONE SERVING FISH AND PEARLED WHEAT IS EQUIVALENT
TO 1½ STARCH + 3 LEAN PROTEIN + 1 FRUIT/LIMITED
VEGETABLE

1 Preheat the oven to 200 °C.

2 Heat the oil in a frying pan and fry the onion and garlic until transparent.

3 Add the curry powder, cinnamon and ginger and fry briefly.

4 Stir the oats and the apricot juice into the onion mixture on the stove. Stir until the mixture thickens and boil briefly. Remove from the stove and set aside.

5 Place the fish in an ovenproof dish and pour the sauce over. Season with salt.

6 Bake for 30 minutes.

7 Boil 190 ml (¾ c) pearled wheat or barley and serve with the fish, and vegetables or salad (e.g. Green bean relish, page 36).

Dietician's notes

• This is a delicious alternative to steamed fish.

• You will notice that, even though we use 190 ml (¾ c) raw pearled wheat, the cooked yield is greater, and the GL lower for the unrefined starches, ie barley, brown rice and pearled wheat. For this reason, rather choose one of these unrefined grains as your starch.

See page 36 for Green bean relish recipe.

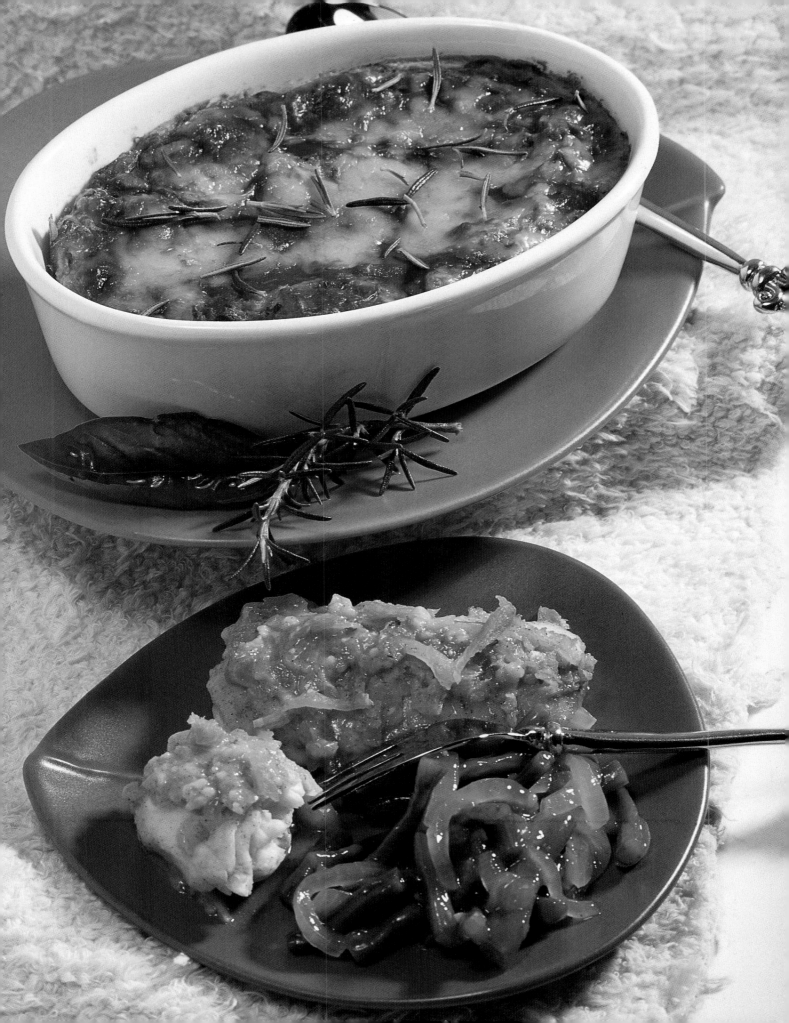

Sweet and sour hake bake

Serves 4

500 g frozen hake fillets
80 ml (scant ⅓ c) low-fat mayonnaise*
1 medium onion, peeled and grated
2 medium green apples, cored and grated
5 ml (1 t) mustard powder
5 ml (1 t) rosemary or thyme
2 ml (½ t) Aromat or other flavour enhancer
45 ml (3 T) lemon juice, freshly squeezed (optional)
a little grated cheese* (optional)

Nutrients per serving (Fish and mash)
Glycaemic Index 54 • Carbohydrates 31 g •
Protein 26 g • Fat 5 g • Fibre 4 g • kJ 1 194 •
Glycaemic load 17

ONE SERVING FISH AND MASH IS EQUIVALENT TO
3 PROTEIN + 1½ STARCH + 1 LIMITED VEGETABLE/
FRUIT

1 Preheat the oven to 200 °C.
2 Place the frozen hake fillets next to each other in an ovenproof dish.
3 Mix the rest of the ingredients, except the cheese, if using, into a thick paste.
4 Spread the sauce over the fish and sprinkle with a little cheese, if desired. Cover and bake for 20 minutes.
5 Remove the cover and bake, uncovered, for another 10 minutes, or until bubbly and lightly browned.
6 Serve with potato and sweet potato mash (2 medium potatoes with 1 medium sweet potato for 4 servings) and 2 cooked vegetables, or salad.

Add zing to the mash with a little mustard or coriander.
If you do not have lemon juice, use apples with a tart flavour.
This sauce is great on leftover chicken, served on a toasted slice of seed loaf.

Dietician's notes

• This is a lovely, tasty low-fat alternative to otherwise bland grilled hake.
• Although Aromat is high in MSG (sodium), so little is used that is will have almost no effect. If you prefer to avoid MSG, use salt instead.

Tuna lasagne

Serves 6

5 ml (1 t) olive oil*
1 large onion, peeled and finely choped
2 cloves garlic, crushed
250 g (1 punnet) mushrooms, wiped clean and sliced
    or 1 x 410 g tin mushrooms (higher in sodium)
200 ml (⅘ c) tomato purée (canned, fresh or in a jar)
    or 4 large tomatoes, chopped
½ x 410 g can baked beans*, mashed
2 x 170 g cans tuna chunks in brine*, drained
15 ml (1 T) soft 'lite' margarine
150 ml (⅗ c) low-fat milk*
125 ml (½ c) water from boiling vegetables
1 ml (¼ t) salt
3 ml (¾ t) mustard powder
45 ml (3 T) flour
5 ml (1 t) finely grated Parmesan
2 ml (½ t) grated nutmeg
160 g (9 sheets) lasagne sheets*
90 g (3 'matchboxes') low-fat cheese*, grated

Nutrients per serving
Glycaemic Index 43 • Carbohydrates 37 g •
Protein 20 g • Fat 7 g • Fibre 4 g • kJ 1 230 •
Glycaemic load 16

ONE SERVING OF LASAGNE IS EQUIVALENT TO
2 STARCH + 2½ PROTEIN + 1 VEGETABLE

1 Heat the oil and gently fry the onion and garlic over moderate heat until the onion is transparent. Add the mushrooms, and stir-fry for 3 minutes.
2 Add the tomato purée or chopped tomatoes and the baked beans. Cook until the sauce thickens. Remove from the stove.
3 Stir in the drained tuna and mix well. Set aside.
4 Make the white sauce. Gently melt the margarine in a small saucepan.
5 Add the milk, the water from boiling the vegetables, the salt and mustard powder. Bring to boil. Meanwhile, mix the flour to a smooth paste with 45 ml water.
6 As soon as the milk boils, pour a little milk onto the flour mixture and stir well until smooth. Pour the flour and water mixture back into the rest of the boiled milk.
7 Return to the heat and boil until the sauce thickens. Remove from the stove.
8 Stir in the Parmesan and the nutmeg.
9 While making the sauce, soak the lasagne sheets in boiling water.
10 Layer a greased 30 x 20 cm lasagne dish with ingredients in this order: some of the pasta, then some of the tuna and tomato sauce, topped with some of the white sauce and a grating of black pepper. Repeat the layers about 3 times.
11 Sprinkle with grated cheese and bake at 200 °C for 20 minutes, or until the cheese bubbles.
12 Alternatively, microwave on high for 10 minutes, or until the cheese bubbles.
13 Serve with a tossed salad.

Please note that this recipe uses uncooked lasagne sheets. If you prefer to use cooked pasta, reduce the water in the white sauce to 80 ml (scant ⅓ c).

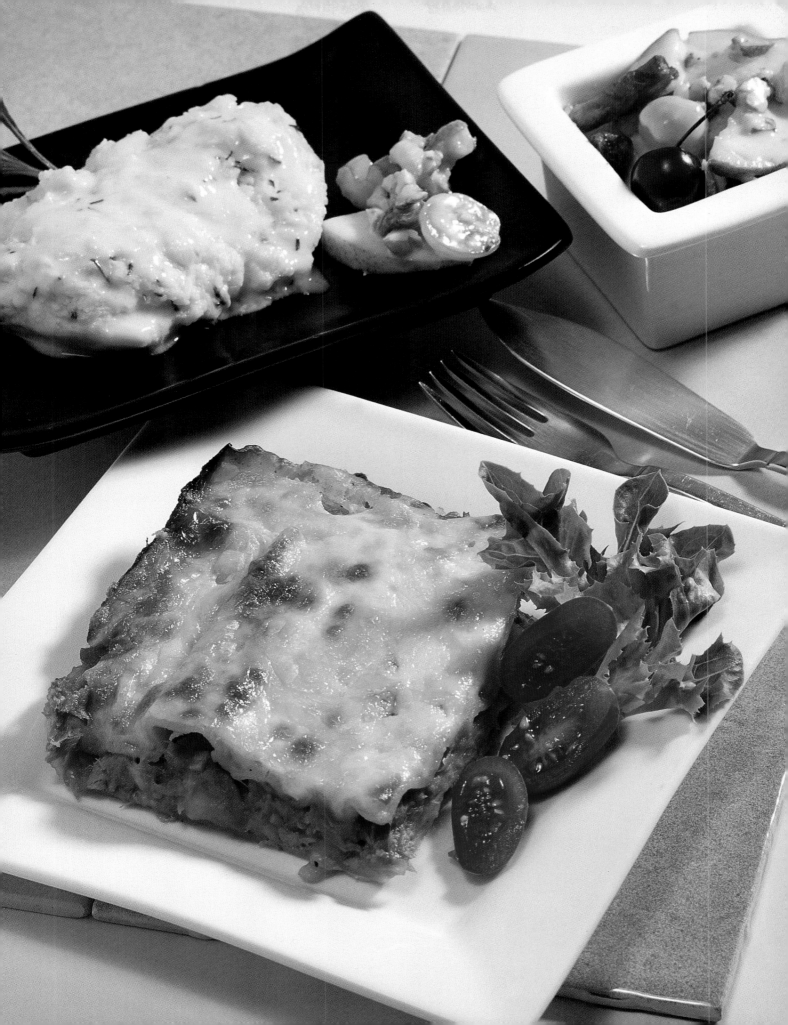

Corn and bean bake

Serves 4

1 x 410 g can butter beans*, drained
1 x 410 g can whole-kernel corn*, drained
    or 250 ml (1 c) cooked corn
5 ml (1 t) oil*
1 large onion, peeled and chopped
2 ml (½ t) salt
250 ml (1 c) skimmed milk*
20 ml (4 t) cornflour
1 ml (¼ t) grated nutmeg
10 ml (2 t) mustard powder
10 ml (2 T) finely grated Parmesan
2 eggs, beaten
freshly ground black pepper to taste
125 ml (½ c) grated mozzarella*
50 ml (⅕ c) chopped parsley
30 g Cheddar cheese, grated (1 'matchbox' of cheese)

Nutrients per serving

Glycaemic Index 40 • Carbohydrates 26 g •
Protein 18 g • Fat 11 g • Fibre 8 g • kJ 1 142 •
Glycaemic load 11

ONE SERVING IS EQUIVALENT TO
1½ STARCH + 2 PROTEIN/DAIRY

1   Preheat the oven to 180 °C.
2   Mix the beans and the corn.
3   Heat the oil in a frying pan and fry the onion until transparent; sprinkle 1 ml (¼ t) of the salt over the fried onions and add to the bean mixture.
4   In a saucepan, heat the milk to boiling point. Mix the cornflour to a smooth paste with 30 ml (2 T) water. Add a little boiled milk to the paste and stir well to make a smooth sauce. Pour the cornflour and milk mixture back into the hot milk in the saucepan, and boil until smooth and thickened, stirring continuously.
5   Add the nutmeg, mustard powder, remaining salt and Parmesan to the white sauce. Mix well. Add the beaten eggs and stir well to mix thoroughly.
6   Mix together the white sauce and the bean mixture. Add the black pepper. Spoon into an ovenproof dish.
7   Sprinkle evenly with the mozzarella, parsley and the Cheddar cheese.
8   Bake for 30 minutes, or until lightly browned.

Any canned dried beans can be used in place of the butter beans.
1 x 410 g can of beans, drained, is equivalent to 250 ml (1 c) cooked dry beans.

Dietician's notes

•   Cheese has a high saturated fat content but lots of flavour, so keep all the cheese for the topping, as this way you get more of a cheese taste. If you mix the cheese into the sauce you lose some of the flavour.
•   Please note how little cheese we used in order to keep the fat content down.

Rice and lentil curry

Serves 4

5 ml (1 t) oil
1 large onion, peeled and chopped
3 cloves garlic, finely chopped or 10 ml (2 t) dried
    garlic flakes
15 ml (1 T) masala (a more aromatic curry powder)
5 ml (1 t) minced chilli
5 ml (1 t) turmeric
2–3 large tomatoes, skinned and chopped
30 ml (2 T) chutney, preferably 'lite'
250 ml (1 c) frozen green peas
500 ml (2 c) cooked lentils or 2 x 410 g cans lentils,
    drained
250 ml (1 c) cooked brown rice
5 ml (1 t) salt
125 ml (½ c) chopped fresh parsley

Nutrients per serving

Glycaemic Index <40 • Carbohydrates 42 g •
Protein 16 g • Fat 2 g • Fibre 13 g • kJ 1 235 •
Glycaemic load 16

ONE SERVING IS EQUIVALENT TO
2 LEAN PROTEIN + 2 STARCH + 2 VEGETABLES

1   Heat the oil in a frying pan and gently fry the onion, garlic and masala.
2   Add the chilli, turmeric, tomatoes and chutney and cook for 10 minutes.
3   Add the peas, cooked lentils, rice and salt; mix and cover.
4   Cook slowly for 10 minutes, until the flavours have combined.
5   Stir in the parsley before serving.

Pasta or any other lower GI rice may be used instead of brown rice.
    Freshly chopped coriander leaves can also be stirred into the curry at the last minute.
    To cook 250 ml (1 c) raw lentils in the microwave, see the recipe for Mushroom and lentil stew on page 68.

Dietician's notes

•   Lentils are a good source of protein, but unlike fish, chicken and (especially) red meat, they contain no fat.
•   This is a complete meal in itself, as it already contains the protein, starch and vegetables of your main meal and the GL is almost at its maximum. There is no need to serve anything with it.
•   Note the exceptionally high fibre content and the low fat content of this meal. That is what happens when lentils are used instead of animal protein.

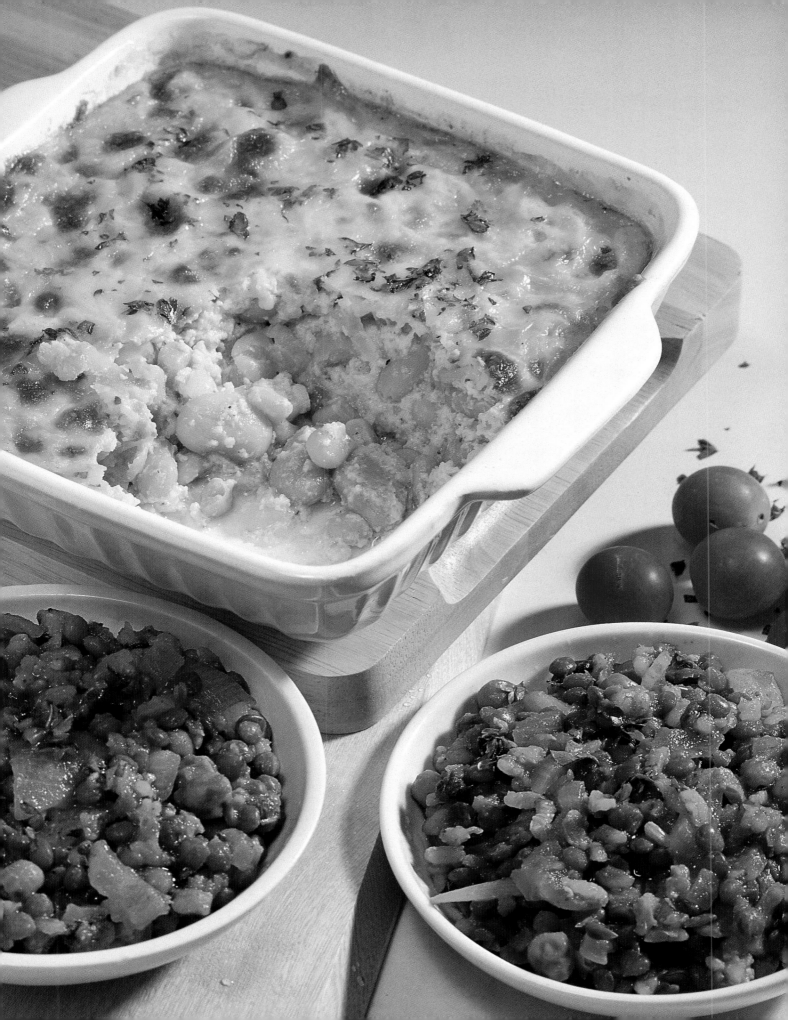

Lentil lasagne

Serves 4

LENTIL SAUCE

10 ml (2 t) olive oil*

1 large onion, peeled and finely chopped

3 cloves garlic, finely chopped

2 ml (½ t) salt

10 ml (2 t) dried mixed herbs

1 tomato, chopped into small cubes

30 ml (2 T) tomato paste

30 ml (2 T) Worcester sauce

15 ml (1 T) sugar

1 carrot, grated

freshly ground black pepper

250 ml (1 c) uncooked split lentils*

WHITE SAUCE

5 ml (1 t) soft 'lite' margarine*

250 ml (1 c) skimmed milk*

45 ml (3 T) oat bran*

30 ml (2 T) flour

1 ml (¼ t) salt

2 ml (½ t) grated nutmeg

120 g (½ box) good-quality durum wheat lasagne
    sheets*

60 g low-fat mozzarella*, grated
    (2 'matchboxes' before grating)

1 Heat the olive oil and gently fry the onion until transparent.

2 Add the garlic and salt. Stir well.

3 Add the herbs and tomato and cook, stirring, until the tomato is mushy.

4 Add the tomato paste, Worcester sauce, sugar, grated carrot, pepper and lentils. Simmer over low heat for 45 minutes. Add water if necessary, as lentils absorb a lot of water.

5 Meanwhile, prepare the white sauce. Melt the margarine in a saucepan over medium heat and let it brown slightly.

6 Pour the milk over the margarine, and bring to the boil.

7 Meanwhile, mix the oat bran, flour, salt and nutmeg with a little water to form a smooth, runny paste.

8 Add to the hot milk and stir over a moderate heat until thick and smooth. Set aside.

9 Preheat the oven to 180 °C.

10 To assemble: Spoon ¼ of the lentil sauce into a lasagne dish and spread out to cover the base. Add 45 ml (3 T) extra 'gravy' to make sure that the first layer of lasagne sheets has adequate liquid in which to cook.

11 Dip each lasagne sheet into hot water and place a single layer of pasta on top of the lentil sauce.

12 Pour ⅓ of the white sauce over the lasagne sheets, spreading it out evenly.

13 Spoon another ¼ of the lentil sauce over this. Continue layering as above, ending with white sauce.

14 Sprinkle with mozzarella and bake for 45 minutes.

15 Serve with a mixed salad.

Dietician's notes

- The analysis alongside is for a whole meal. Adding a tossed salad with a low-oil dressing will raise the kilojoule count slightly and bring the GL up to 28, which is quite acceptable for a main meal, considering the GI is so low.

- Note the exceptionally high fibre content so typical of vegetarian meals containing legumes (lentils).

- This meal should keep you full for at least 4–5 hours … a perfect main meal lunch for a long afternoon of meetings or rushing around with children, or an afternoon of sport. Make the lasagne the day before, and simply reheat it for lunch the next day.

- Please note that the Glycaemic load of most low GI main meals (such as those in this book), is in the vicinity of 20. This means that three meals per day should add up to a GL of between 60 and 70, leaving 30 GL points for snacks and drinks. The aim is to keep the total GL per day under 100.

Nutrients per serving

Glycaemic Index 40 • Carbohydrates 65 g •
Protein 26 g • Fat 8 g • Fibre 13 g • kJ 1 841 •
Glycaemic load 26

ONE SERVING OF LASAGNE IS EQUIVALENT TO
2½ STARCH + 3 PROTEIN/DAIRY + VEGETABLE

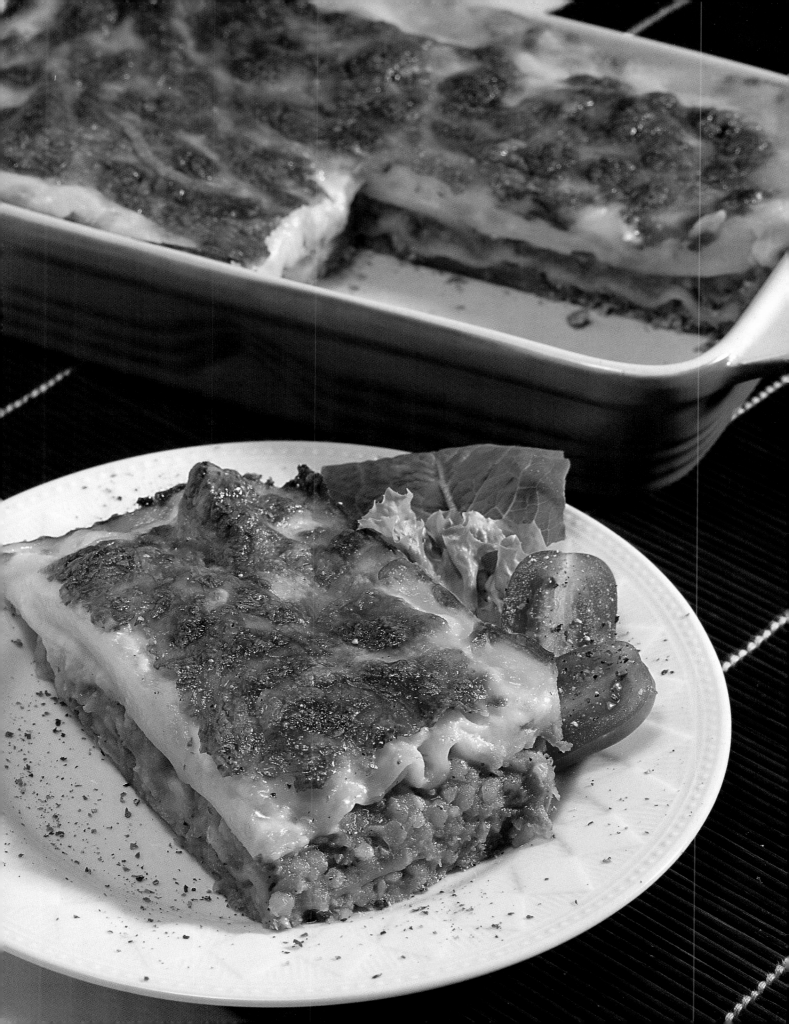

Mushroom and lentil stew

Serves 4

10 ml (2 t) olive oil*

1 large onion, peeled and chopped

2 cloves of garlic, crushed

1 carrot, peeled and grated

1 sweet red pepper, seeded and chopped

500 ml (2 c) cooked lentils* or 2 x 410 g cans lentils, drained*

300 g brown mushrooms, sliced

30 ml (2 T) tomato paste

2 ml (½ t) sugar

100 ml (⅖ c) chopped fresh parsley

2 ml (½ t) dried basil or 30 ml (2 T) chopped fresh basil leaves

2 ml (½ t) dried thyme or 30 ml (2 T) chopped fresh thyme

5 ml (1 t) vegetable stock powder

125 ml (½ c) hot water

salt and freshly ground black pepper to taste

Nutrients per serving

Glycaemic Index 29 • Carbohydrates 29 g •
Protein 14 g • Fat 3 g • Fibre 13 g • kJ 833 •
Glycaemic load 8

ONE SERVING IS EQUIVALENT TO
1 STARCH + 1½ PROTEIN + VEGETABLES

1   Heat the oil in a large saucepan and fry the onion and garlic until transparent.
2   Add the carrot, red pepper and lentils, and stir-fry for 2 minutes.
3   Add the mushrooms, tomato paste, sugar, parsley, basil, thyme, stock powder and hot water. Cover and simmer for 15 minutes, or until the vegetables are tender.
4   Season with a little salt (salt is only needed if freshly cooked lentils are used; canned lentils are already salted) and freshly ground black pepper.
5   Serve hot, garnished with strips of sundried tomato or red pepper, together with a large mixed salad and a fruit for pudding.

This dish is particularly tasty if you use fresh herbs instead of dried. The parsley also adds lots of colour.

To cook lentils quickly, add 250 ml (1 c) lentils to 500 ml (2 c) boiling water and microwave on high for 5 minutes. Drain off the water and add another 250 ml (1 c) of boiling water. Microwave on high for 12 minutes. Voilà! Cooked lentils ready to add to any vegetarian dish.

Dietician's notes

*   Note the exceptionally high fibre content, because of the lentils. This is typical of many vegetarian dishes containing legumes.
*   This is a lighter meal than lentil lasagne, so you could have a starch-containing snack, e.g. 1 biscuit or rusk (see pages 112–118) later on, or one of the puddings (pages 86–94).
*   Usually we recommend using only 5 ml (1 t) oil for fake-frying, but in this recipe we used 10 ml (2 t) as it is the only fat in the dish.

Cabbage stir-fry

Serves 4

5 ml (1 t) olive or canola oil*

1 medium onion, peeled and chopped

400 g cabbage, shredded or 1 litre (4 c) shredded cabbage (¼ cabbage)

5 ml (1 t) chicken stock powder

1   Heat the oil in a frying pan.
2   Stir-fry the onion until transparent.
3   Add the cabbage and fry until lightly browned. Stir frequently.
4   Sprinkle the stock powder over the cabbage, mix well and fry a little longer.
5   Serve on its own, or with a low-fat cheese sauce (page 76) as an accompaniment to a main meal.

Stock powder may be used instead of salt in many dishes. It adds flavour without too much sodium; it contains ⅓ less sodium than salt.

Dietician's notes

*   This is a welcome alternative to boiled cabbage.
*   You will notice that the GL of this vegetable dish is very low, which implies that it cannot lower the GI of high GI starches like potatoes (which also have a high GL). It also implies that it has very little effect on the GI of the meal and thus almost no effect on blood glucose levels.
*   Eat with a meal containing a low GI starch.

See page 76 for white sauce recipe (pictured with the Cabbage stir-fry).

Nutrients per serving

Glycaemic Index < 40 • Carbohydrates 6 g •
Protein 2 g • Fat 1 g • Fibre 3 g • kJ 205 •
Glycaemic load 1

ONE SERVING IS EQUIVALENT TO
1 VEGETABLE

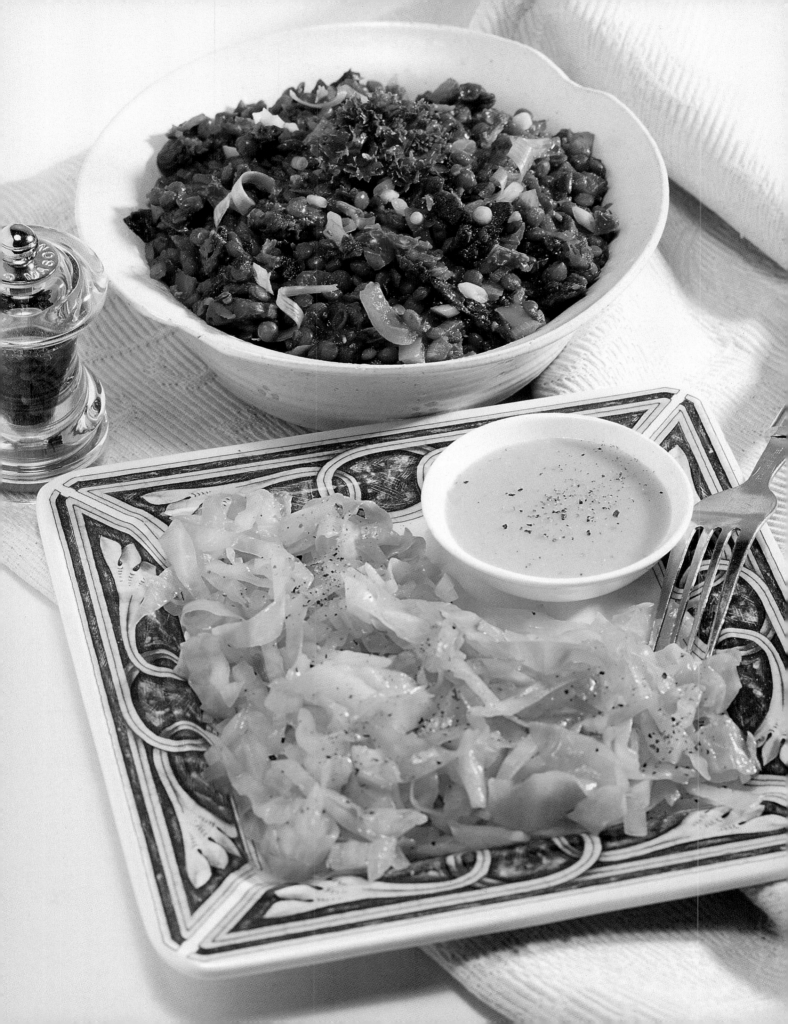

Napolitana sauce for pasta

Serves 4

5 ml (1 t) canola or olive oil*

2 medium onions, peeled and chopped

5 ml (1 t) crushed garlic or 2 cloves garlic, chopped

1 carrot, peeled and grated coarsely

½ sweet green pepper, chopped

4 ripe tomatoes, peeled and diced

5 ml (1 t) dried thyme

5 ml (1 t) dried origanum

5 ml (1 t) dried basil

2 ml (½ t) salt

freshly ground black pepper to taste

1 x 65–70 g can tomato paste

½ x 410 g can butter beans*, drained and mashed

20 ml (4 t) grated Parmesan

> **Nutrients per serving**
>
> (sauce and pasta)
>
> Glycaemic Index <40 • Carbohydrates 47 g •
> Protein 12 g • Fats 4 g • Fibre 9 g • kJ 1 265 •
> Glycaemic load 17
>
> ONE SERVING OF PASTA AND SAUCE IS EQUIVALENT TO
> 2 STARCH +1 PROTEIN + 2 VEGETABLES

1 Heat the oil in a large saucepan and gently fry the onions, garlic, carrot and green pepper until the onions are transparent. If they start to burn, add 15–30 ml (1–2 T) of water and stir.
2 Add the diced tomatoes and simmer for 5 minutes.
3 Add the herbs, salt, pepper, tomato paste and mashed beans, and simmer for a further 5 minutes.
4 Spoon over freshly cooked pasta of your choice (use ⅓ x 500 g packet for 4 servings) on a serving dish and sprinkle with Parmesan.
5 Serve immediately with either cooked vegetables or a tossed salad.

For a mushroom sauce for pasta see page 121.

Dietician's notes

- This meal is ideal for carbo-loading as it contains long-acting carbohydrates with not too much fat and protein.
- The GI of carrots is generally high, but in this recipe, combined with the beans and other low GI vegetables, its effect is cancelled out.
- Note the exceptionally high fibre content; good for lowering cholesterol and controlling blood glucose levels.

Creamy vegetable sauce for pasta

Serves 4

5 ml (1 t) canola or olive oil*

2 small onions, peeled and chopped

10 ml (2 t) minced garlic

250 g (1 punnet) sliced mushrooms

½ sweet green pepper, chopped

1 carrot, peeled and grated

250 ml (1 c) broccoli, cut into small florets

1 x 410 g can baked beans in tomato sauce*, mashed

15 ml (1 T) tomato purée

5 ml (1 t) dried mixed herbs

125 ml (½ c) low-fat milk*

pinch of grated nutmeg

2 ml (½ t) salt

freshly ground black pepper to taste

> **Nutrients per serving**
>
> Glycaemic Index 40 • Carbohydrates 57 g •
> Protein 15 g • Fat 5 g • Fibre 14 g • kJ 1 426 •
> Glycaemic load 23
>
> ONE SERVING OF PASTA AND SAUCE IS EQUIVALENT TO
> 1½ PROTEIN + 2½ STARCH + 2 VEGETABLES

1 Heat the oil in a nonstick frying pan. Add the onions and garlic, and cook for about 5 minutes.
2 Add the mushrooms, green pepper and carrot. Cook for a further 5 minutes.
3 Add the broccoli, baked beans, tomato purée and herbs.
4 Stir in the milk and nutmeg.
5 Simmer for 15 minutes.
6 Once the sauce has thickened slightly, season it with salt and pepper.
7 Serve on freshly cooked pasta of your choice (use ⅓ x 500 g packet for 4 servings).

Butter beans or kidney beans may be used instead of baked beans. Use 250 ml (1 c) cooked dried kidney beans or 1 x 410 g can butter beans, drained.
The tomato purée can be left out if you prefer a whiter sauce.

Dietician's notes

- This dish has an exceptionally high fibre content and is also very low in fat.
- Since the beans are mashed in this sauce, it is also ideal for those suffering from irritable bowel syndrome.
- A Glycaemic load of 23 is ideal for a main meal, especially with a low GI of 40 – enjoy!

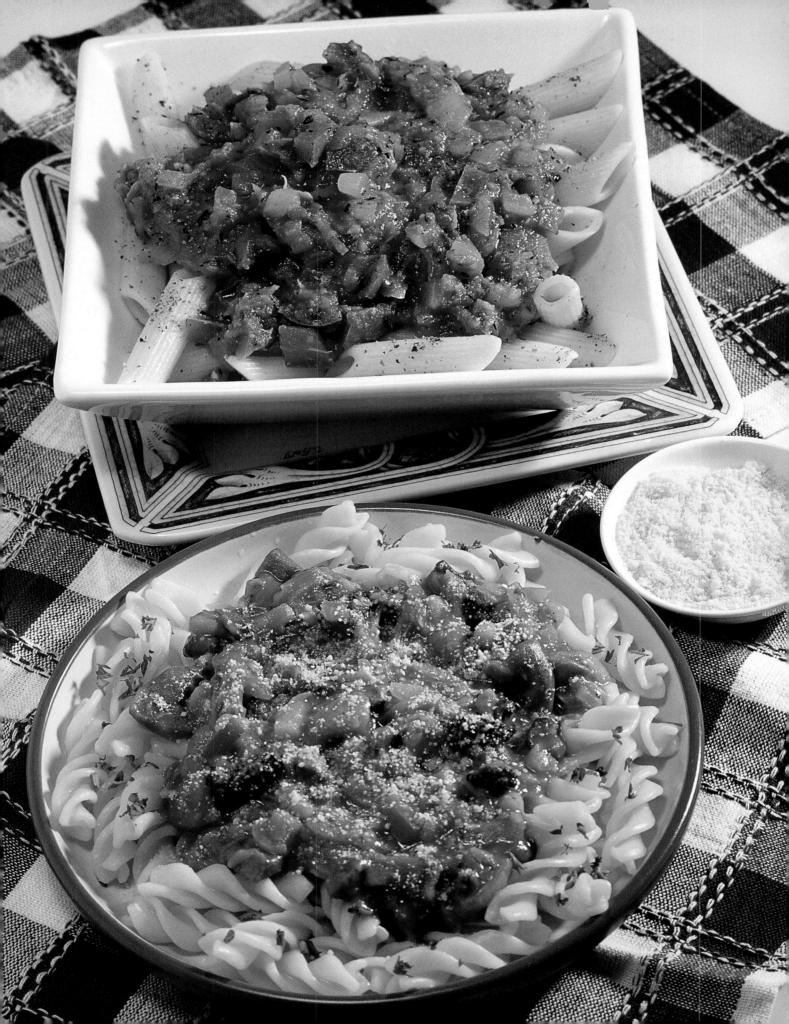

Gourmet green beans

Serves 4

5 ml (1 t) canola or olive oil*
1 small onion, peeled and chopped
2 rashers bacon*, chopped, fat discarded (30 g
    uncooked)
500 ml (2 c) frozen green beans or 1 x 410 g can green
    beans, drained

1   Heat the oil and fry the onion until transparent.
2   Add the bacon and fry until browned, stirring occasionally.
3   Add the green beans and fry until heated through and lightly browned.

If you prefer to use fresh green beans, you will need 350 g. Wash, top and tail the green beans, and cut them into 2 cm long pieces. Boil the beans in 125 ml (½ c) water for 10 minutes to soften, then use the beans as directed above.

Dietician's notes

- This is a tasty way to serve green beans.
- Prepared like this, the beans can also be used to fill butternut (see Stuffed butternut recipe below), and in so doing the beans lower the GI of the higher GI butternut.
- Please note that the GL of most vegetables is below 5, which means that vegetables not only add vitamins and minerals to a meal, but also help to keep the Glycaemic Index and Glycaemic load of the meal in check.

Nutrients per serving

Glycaemic Index <40 • Carbohydrates 5 g •
Protein 3 g • Fat 2 g • Fibre 2 g • kJ 224 •
Glycaemic load 2

ONE SERVING IS EQUIVALENT TO
1 VEGETABLE + ½ FAT

Stuffed butternut

Serves 4

4 small butternuts or 1 medium butternut
1 recipe Gourmet green beans (above)
½ feta round* (40 g)

1   Preheat the oven to 200 °C.
2   If you are using 4 small butternuts, cut off the necks of the butternuts and reserve the flesh for use in another dish. Use the 4 bodies as cups to be filled. Remove the pips and boil or microwave until soft/cooked.
3   If using 1 medium butternut, slice it lengthways and halve each section to make 4 portions. Hollow out the necks and remove the pips.
4   Prepare Gourmet green beans as described above, but crumble half of the feta onto the beans towards the end of the cooking process. Stir until the feta has just melted.
5   Fill the butternut cups or quarters with the green bean mixture. Crumble the rest of the feta on top of the green bean mixture in the butternut cups.
6   Bake in the oven until the cheese has melted.
7   Serve with a main meal, e.g. Unbelievable chicken (page 48).

This is an extraordinary way of serving both butternut and green beans, and is a dish to impress your guests!
    Feta cheese with black pepper is particularly tasty in this dish.

Dietician's notes

- This is an ideal way of lowering higher GI butternut with lower GI green beans.
- Note that the GL is low in spite of the high GI butternut. This is because vegetables do not contain large quantities of carbohydrates, so all vegetables (high and low GI) can be included in every meal.
- Note the high fibre content per serving of these vegetables.
- Remember that this vegetable dish does contain fat (from the cheese and oil from the gourmet green beans), so compensate for this by ensuring that other dishes in the meal are lower in fat.

Nutrients per serving

Glycaemic Index 57 • Carbohydrates 13 g •
Protein 5 g • Fat 5 g • Fibre 5 g • kJ 551 •
Glycaemic load 8

ONE SERVING IS EQUIVALENT TO
2 LIMITED VEGETABLE + 1 FAT

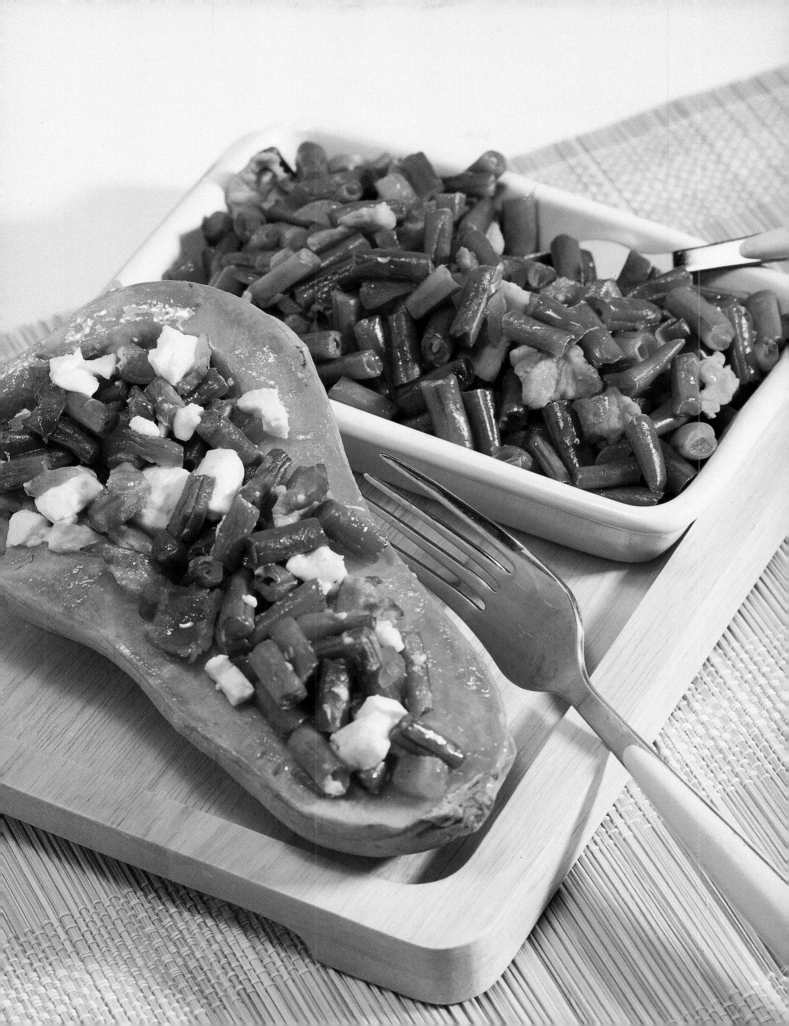

Roast vegetables
Serves 6

200 g butternut, peeled, cubed (½ large butternut)
30 ml (2 T) oil*
1 clove garlic, crushed, or more, if you are fond
  of garlic
5 ml (1 t) vegetable stock powder dissolved in 80 ml
  (scant ⅓ c) hot water
30 ml (2 T) raw honey
3 courgettes, cut into 3 cm pieces
6 patty pans, cut into quarters
250 g mixed baby veggies (625 ml [2½ c])
20 cherry tomatoes
250 g (about 16) button mushrooms
freshly ground black pepper to taste (optional)

Nutrients per serving

Glycaemic Index 49 • Carbohydrates 12 g •
Protein 3 g • Fat 5 g • Fibre 4 g • kJ 445 •
Glycaemic load 6

ONE SERVING OF ROAST VEGETABLES IS EQUIVALENT TO
2 VEGETABLE + ½ FAT

ONE SERVING OF ROAST VEGETABLES WITH CHEESE AND
OLIVES IS EQUIVALENT TO 2 VEGETABLE + 1 PROTEIN
+ ½ FAT

1   Preheat the oven to 200 °C.
2   Boil or steam the butternut until almost soft.
3   Pour the oil into a baking tray and heat it in the oven.
4   Mix the garlic, dissolved stock powder, and honey and set aside.
5   Add all the vegetables to the hot baking tray and turn to coat with the oil.
6   Drizzle the honey mixture over the vegetables.
7   Cover and bake for 20–30 minutes, turning the vegetables twice.
8   Grill, uncovered, for a few minutes before serving, if desired.
9   Serve with black pepper, if desired.

Variation: For more of an Italian flavour, leave out the oil and add 8 olives and 120 g (4 'matchboxes') lower fat white cheese pressed into chopped basil, at the end of the baking time, then place the tray under a hot grill for 3 minutes to just melt the cheese. Sprinkle with a little balsamic vinegar, if desired.

Any vegetables may be used as long as you end up with 1 kg chopped vegetables.

If you do not want to bake the dish for the full 20 minutes, parcook all the vegetables and the dish will only need 10 minutes in a hot oven or under the grill.

Dietician's notes

•   Note that, in spite of the higher GI honey and butternut, the GL of this dish is low because it is purely vegetable.
•   Remember, if you make the Italian version, that the cheese contributes protein and fat to the meal, so compensate by having a smaller portion of protein in this meal. Do not forget to omit the oil.

Roast sweet potatoes and butternut
Serves 4

2 medium sweet potatoes (at least 200 g each)
½ small butternut, peeled and diced (not more than
  200 g)
15 ml (1 T) canola or olive oil*
5 ml (1 t) dried or fresh rosemary or 10 ml (2t)
  cinnamon sugar

1   Cook the sweet potatoes and butternut until just done, but still firm.
2   Meanwhile, preheat the oven to 200 °C.
3   Peel the sweet potatoes and cut into large chunks.
4   Pour oil into a flat baking pan and place the pan into the hot oven.
5   As soon as the oil is hot, about 5 minutes, remove the baking pan from the oven, swirl it to make sure the base is covered with oil, then pour all the oil out.
6   Place the cooked sweet potatoes and butternut in the baking pan and toss or turn until all the vegetables are completely covered in a thin layer of oil.
7   Sprinkle with the rosemary or cinnamon sugar, if desired.
8   Roast, turning once, until evenly browned.
9   Serve with a salad and a small portion of lean, grilled meat, fish or chicken.

Dietician's notes

•   Even those with diabetes you can use the cinnamon sugar option; at only 2 g sugar per serving, it will have a negligible effect on blood glucose levels.
•   Potatoes have a high GI, but sweet potatoes have a low GI. For this reason we have included a low-fat method of roasting sweet potatoes.
•   Butternut has not been tested for its GI, but because the only internationally tested GI values we have for yellow pumpkin are high, it would be best that the quantity of butternut you use is half that of the sweet potato (note the quantities in the recipe).

Nutrients per serving

Glycaemic Index 56 • Carbohydrates 27 g •
Protein 2 g • Fat 2 g • Fibre 5 g • kJ 621 •
Glycaemic load 15

ONE SERVING IS EQUIVALENT TO
1½ STARCH + 1 LIMITED VEGETABLE

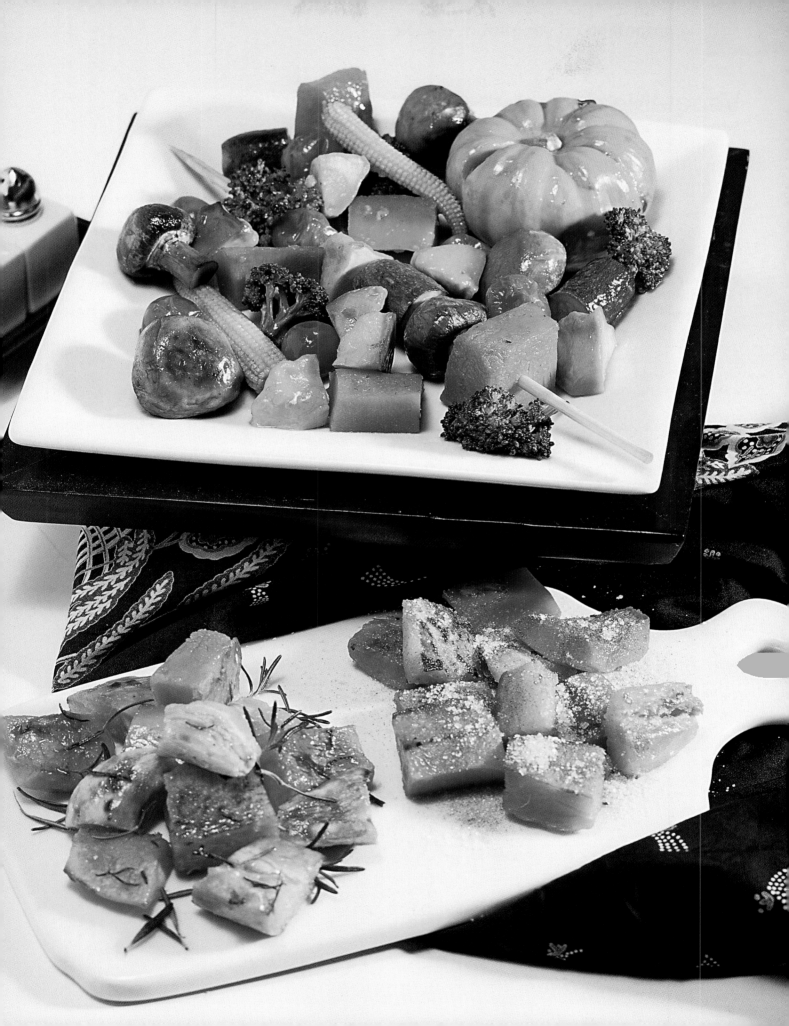

Vegetable duos with white sauce
Serves 4

Cauliflower and Broccoli

300 g cauliflower florets

300 g broccoli florets

WHITE SAUCE

15 ml (1 T) soft 'lite' margarine*

45 ml (3 T) flour

125 ml (½ c) water reserved from boiling vegetables,
   or chicken or vegetable stock, or 5 ml (1 t) stock
   powder dissolved in 125 ml (½ c) boiling water

2–3 cloves garlic, finely chopped or 5–7 ml (1–1 ½ t)
   dried garlic flakes

185 ml (¾ cup) skimmed or low-fat milk

1 ml (¼ t) salt (optional)

30 g lower fat cheese* (preferably yellow)

1 Boil the cauliflower and broccoli in half their weight of boiling water (125 ml [½ c] water to 250 ml [1 c] vegetables) until tender, but not too soft. Drain and keep the cooking liquid to use as vegetable stock.
2 Make the sauce. In a medium saucepan, melt the margarine and add the flour. Stir until the mixture resembles soft crumbs.
3 Gradually add the vegetable water or stock, and the garlic, stirring continuously with a whisk to make a smooth sauce.
4 Add the milk, stirring continuously, and cook gently until the sauce thickens.
5 Lastly, add the salt, if desired.
6 Place the cauliflower and broccoli in a dish and pour over the white sauce. Grate the cheese on top.
8 Serve with any main meal, especially those containing only 2 portions of protein e.g. Chili con carne (page 78).

Nutrients per portion

Glycaemic Index 40 • Carbohydrates 11 g •
Protein 8 g • Fat 3 g • Fibre 4 g • kJ 471 •
Glycaemic load 4

ONE SERVING IS EQUIVALENT TO
1 DAIRY + 2 VEGETABLES

Dietician's notes

- Omit the salt in the white sauce if stock powder was used to make the stock.
- Brussels sprouts can be used instead of broccoli. The fibre content would then double.
- The cheese adds extra protein (and kilojoules) to this variation of white sauce.
- Note that the nutritional analysis was done using skimmed fat-free milk.

Courgettes and mushrooms

5 ml (1 t) oil*

1 medium onion, peeled and chopped

1–3 cloves garlic, finely chopped,
   or 5–7 ml (1–1½ t) dried garlic flakes

200 g (about 6) courgettes (baby marrows), chopped

250 g mushrooms, chopped

WHITE SAUCE

15 ml (1 T) soft 'lite' margarine*

45 ml (3 T) flour

125 ml (½ c) water reserved from boiling vegetables,
   or chicken or vegetable stock, or 5 ml (1 t) stock
   powder dissolved in 125 ml (½ cup) boiling water

185 ml (¾ cup) skimmed or low-fat milk

1 ml (¼ t) salt (optional)

lots of black pepper

1 Heat the oil in a frying pan and fry the onions and garlic until transparent.
2 Add the mushrooms and courgettes and stir-fry, but do not overcook. Remove from the heat and pour off the excess liquid, or keep it as 'stock' for the white sauce. Set aside.
3 Make the sauce. In a medium saucepan, melt the margarine and add the flour. Stir until the mixture resembles soft crumbs. Gradually add the water from cooking the vegetables, or the stock, stirring continuously with a whisk to make a smooth sauce.
5 Add the milk, stirring continuously, and cook gently until the sauce thickens.
6 Add salt (if desired) and black pepper to taste.
7 Serve the vegetables topped with the white sauce, or mix the vegetables with the white sauce before serving.

Nutrients per serving

Glycaemic Index 40 • Carbohydrates 13 g •
Protein 4 g • Fat 3 g • Fibre 2 g • kJ 429 •
Glycaemic load 5

ONE SERVING IS EQUIVALENT TO
½ DAIRY + 1 VEGETABLE

Dietician's notes

- Omit the salt in the white sauce if stock powder was used to make the stock.
- Please note that the nutritional analysis was done using skimmed fat-free milk.

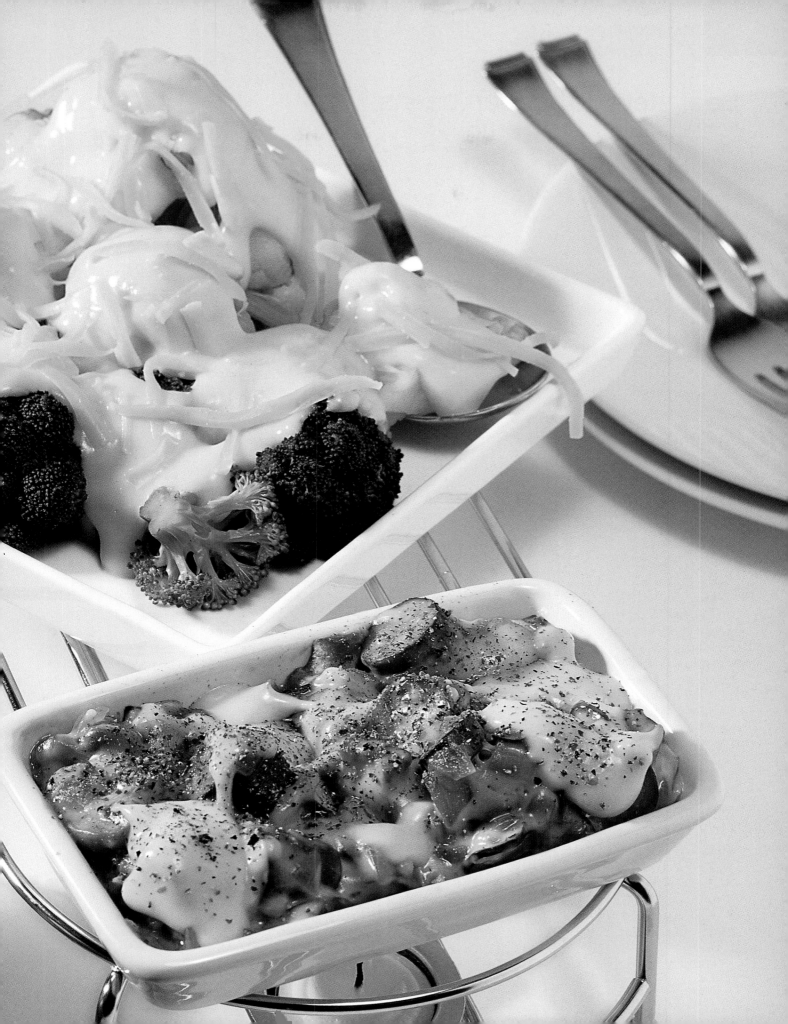

Beef stew with green beans

Serves 4

5 ml (1 t) oil*
2 rashers lean bacon*, chopped, fat discarded
1 large onion, peeled and diced
2 ml (½ t) garlic flakes or 1 clove garlic, chopped
400 g goulash meat, cubed, fat discarded
15 ml (1 T) Worcester sauce
1 ml (¼ t) paprika
1 ml (¼ t) ground cloves
freshly ground black pepper to taste
10 ml (2 t) beef stock powder
250 ml (1 c) frozen green beans or 500 ml (2 c) uncooked raw green beans or 1 x 410 g can sliced green beans, drained
30 ml (2 T) lower GI oats*

Nutrients per serving (Stew and rice)
Glycaemic Index 46 • Carbohydrates 35 g •
Protein 30 g • Fat 8 g • Fibre 2 g • kJ 1 386 •
Glycaemic load 16

ONE SERVING OF STEW AND RICE IS EQUIVALENT TO
3 PROTEIN + 1½ STARCH + VEGETABLE

1 Heat the oil in a large saucepan; add the bacon, onion and garlic, and gently fry until the onion is transparent.
2 Add the meat, Worcester sauce, spices, pepper and stock powder. Fry for 5–10 minutes, stirring frequently.
3 Add the green beans and oats and simmer, with the lid on, for another 20–30 minutes. Add water as needed if the stew gets too thick.
4 Serve with lower GI rice (boil 185 ml [¾ c] uncooked rice to serve 4), vegetables and salad, e.g. cooked butternut and a tomato salad.

This is a really tasty old-fashioned stew, perfect for those cold winter nights.
   Add a little balsamic vinegar and sugar (optional) to the tomato salad to give it an extra-special taste.

Dietician's notes

* The effect of the higher GI butternut is balanced out by the lower GI green beans, oats, tomato salad and rice.
* The nutritional analysis is for the stew with the rice. The stew on its own has an insignificant GI and GL, due to the small quantity of carbohydrate it contains.
* Women may prefer to have only one starch portion; if so, dish up a little more rice for the men.

Chilli con carne

Serves 10

5 ml (1 t) oil*
2 medium onions, peeled and chopped
2 cloves garlic, crushed
500 g lean topside mince
2 sweet green peppers, chopped
15 ml (1 T) ground coriander
5 ml (1 t) ground cinnamon
10 ml (2 t) cumin seed (optional)
2 ml (½ t) dried origanum
2 ml (½ t) dried mixed herbs
45 ml (3 T) chopped fresh parsley
20–25 ml (4–5 t) chilli powder, or to taste
2 ml (½ t) salt
1 x 65 g can tomato paste
100 ml (⅖ c) water
1½ x 410 g cans baked beans in tomato sauce*
5 pita breads (½ per person)

Nutrients per serving (with ½ pita bread)
Glycaemic Index 50 • Carbohydrates 43 g •
Protein 19 g • Fat 6 g • Fibre 8 g • kJ 1 262 •
Glycaemic load 22

ONE SERVING IS EQUIVALENT TO
2½ STARCH + 2 LEAN PROTEIN

1 Heat the oil in a large saucepan and gently fry the onions and garlic, stirring continuously, until the onions are transparent.
2 Add the minced meat and fry until browned.
3 Add the green peppers, spices, herbs, chilli, salt, and freshly ground black pepper to taste.
4 Stir in the tomato paste and water and simmer for 20 minutes. Stir occasionally.
5 Add the baked beans and heat through.
6 Serve in half a pita bread per person. Split the half pita and overfill with chilli con carne, add a salad with a low-oil dressing and you have a balanced meal.
7 Alternatively, serve with rice (500 ml [2 c] uncooked rice to serve 10) and salad.

Dietician's notes

* One pita pocket is equivalent to 3 slices of bread, so we suggest you only use half a pita pocket per person.
* The pita bread has a marked effect on the GI and the Glycaemic load of this meal because it is so dense in carbohydrates.
* This chilli con carne makes a very filling meal and, because we use the low-fat method of preparation, the fat content of the meal is well below the recommended 10–13 g of fat for the whole meal.
* This meal probably contains a bit more starch than most would like, but as the protein is slightly less, it will balance out.

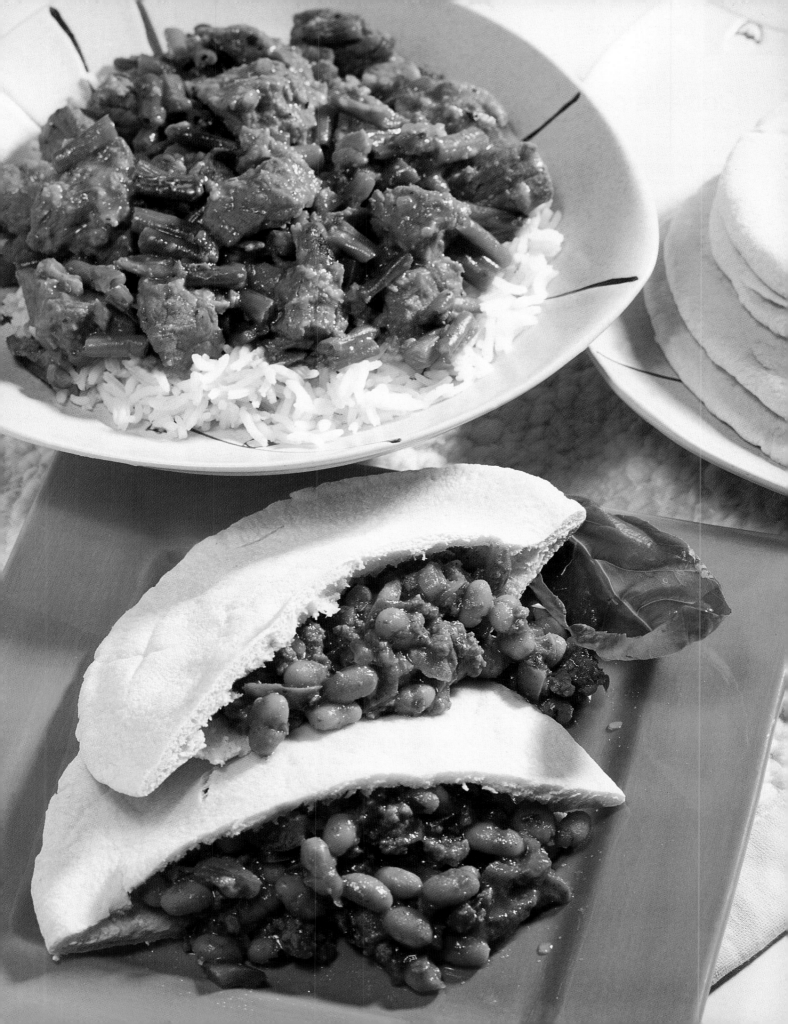

Cottage pie
Serves 4

5 ml (1 t) olive or canola oil*

1 medium onion, peeled and chopped

1 clove garlic, crushed or 2 ml (½ t) garlic flakes

300 g topside mince

5 ml (1 t) beef stock powder or ¼ beef stock cube

30 ml (2 T) chopped fresh or 2 ml (½ t) dried parsley

2 ml (½ t) dried mixed herbs

freshly ground black pepper

15 ml (1 T) Worcester sauce

1 x 410 g can baked beans in tomato sauce*

TOPPING

300 g (1 large or 2 medium) potatoes

60 ml (4 T) skimmed milk*

5 ml (1 t) baking powder

30 g lower fat cheese*, grated (1 'matchbox' cheese before grating)

paprika

Nutrients per serving

Glycaemic Index 59 • Carbohydrates 36 g •
Protein 25 g • Fat 9 g • Fibre 10 g • kJ 1 399 •
Glycaemic load 21

ONE SERVING IS EQUIVALENT TO
3 PROTEIN + 2 STARCH

---

1 Preheat the oven to 180 °C.
2 Heat the oil and fry the onion and garlic until the onion is transparent.
3 Add the mince, stock powder or stock cube, herbs and pepper, and stir-fry for 5–10 minutes to brown the mince.
4 Add the Worcester sauce and baked beans, and cook for another 5–10 minutes.
5 Spoon into a lightly greased ovenproof dish.
6 Make the topping. Peel the potatoes and boil until just soft.
7 Add the milk and baking powder, and mash the potatoes until light and fluffy.
8 Spread the mashed potatoes over the mince mixture in the ovenproof dish.
9 Sprinkle first the cheese and then the paprika on top.
10 Bake for 20 minutes, or until heated through and bubbling.
11 Serve with vegetables only, e.g. 1 of the vegetable duos (page 76), as 1 portion of cottage pie already contains your protein and starch.

Dietician's notes

• Even though we have reduced the mash to only 300 g for 4 people, and added low GI baked beans to the mince, the GI of this cottage pie is still above 55. However, if you layer cooked baby potatoes on top of the mince instead of mash, the GI drops to 51 (and the GL becomes 18). The moral of the story? Potato is a dense, high GI food, with a high GL as well. This means that potatoes have a substantial impact on blood glucose levels.
• Remember to use lower fat cheese and skimmed milk, and don't use any more oil than stated, as the fat content is already quite high.
• As soon as red meat is included in a recipe, the fat content shoots up.
• Note the high fibre content. This is due to the baked beans in the meat.

Chutney chops
Serves 4

2 small lamb chops or 1 large lamb chop per person

SAUCE

45 ml (3 T) chutney, preferably 'lite'

15 ml (1 T) vinegar

2 ml (½ t) Aromat (use sparingly – it is high in sodium)

5 ml (1 t) mustard powder

5 ml (1 t) dried herbs or 15 ml (1 T) fresh herbs of your choice (mint works well)

Nutrients per serving
(Including the sweet potato and butternut)
Glycaemic Index 55 • Carbohydrates 32 g •
Protein 30 g • Fat 10 g • Fibre 5 g • kJ 1 511 •
Glycaemic load 18

ONE SERVING (CHOPS, SWEET POTATO AND BUTTERNUT)
IS EQUIVALENT TO 3 PROTEIN, 1½ STARCH AND
1 LIMITED VEGETABLE

---

1 Preheat the oven to 200 °C.
2 Remove all visible fat from the lamb chops.
3 Place the chops in a lightly greased ovenproof dish and place in the oven.
4 Prepare a sauce by mixing the rest of the ingredients together.
5 Turn the chops after about 15 minutes and spread with half of the sauce on the turned up side. Save some of the sauce for the other side. Bake until browned, 10–15 minutes.
6 Turn the chops again and spread the rest of the sauce on the other side. Bake until browned, 5–10 minutes.
7 Serve immediately with Roast sweet potatoes and butternut (page 74), as well as 2 other vegetables.

Please note: Use 15 ml (1 T) extra vinegar if ordinary chutney is used, otherwise the sauce will be too thick and too little to cover all the chops.

Dietician's notes

• Lamb and mutton are the fattiest of all meats. The fat content of this meal can be reduced even further by cooking the chops on an oven rack and placing an ovenproof dish below the rack, so that all the marbled fat can drip into the ovenproof dish as the chops cook. Discard this fat.
• This recipe lends itself very well to braaiing.

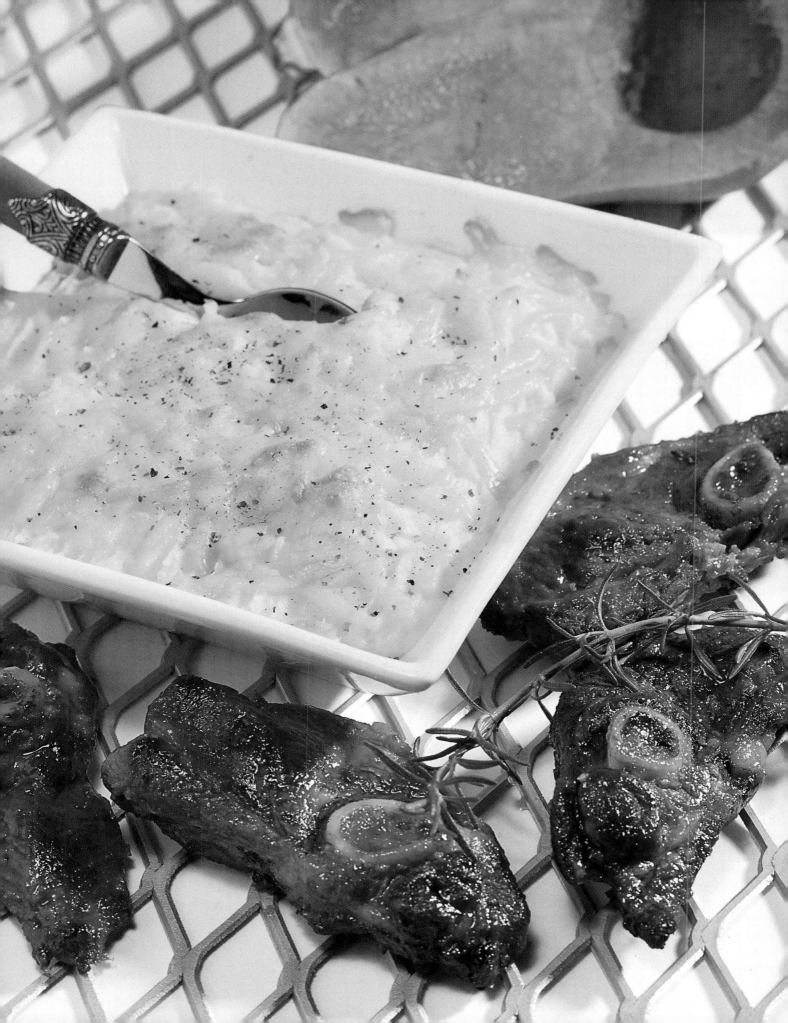

Glazed meat loaf (Microwave recipe)

Serves 8

125 ml (½ c) skimmed milk*
125 ml (½ c) lower GI oats*
2 ml (½ t) salt
2 ml (½ t) dried sage
2 eggs
5 ml (1 t) Worcester sauce
1 large onion, peeled and chopped
60 ml (4 T) finely chopped sweet green pepper
30 ml (2 T) finely chopped fresh parsley
450 g lean minced beef
1 x 410 g can lentils, or 250 ml (1 c) cooked lentils*
75 ml (5 T) tomato sauce
30 ml (2 T) brown sugar
5 ml (1 t) Dijon mustard
dash of grated nutmeg

Nutrients per serving
(Meat loaf and sweetcorn)
Glycaemic Index 57 • Carbohydrates 37 g •
Protein 18 g • Fat 7 g • Fibre 7 g • kJ 1 183 •
Glycaemic load 19

ONE SERVING OF MEAT LOAF AND SWEETCORN IS
EQUIVALENT TO 2 STARCH + 2½ PROTEIN

1 Pour the milk over the oats and leave to stand while gathering together the rest of the ingredients.
2 Place the salt, sage, eggs, Worcester sauce and onion in a large bowl. Add the green pepper, parsley, beef, drained lentils, freshly ground black pepper to taste and soaked oats, and mix well.
3 Pat the mixture evenly into a 23 cm x 13 cm rectangular glass microwave dish.
4 Stir together the tomato sauce, sugar, mustard and nutmeg and spread evenly over the top of the meat loaf.
5 Microwave on high for 18–20 minutes, or until cooked to your preference.
6 Allow to stand for at least 5 minutes before serving.
7 To serve, cut into slices and add 2 cooked vegetables or a salad and a low GI starch, e.g. green mealies or sweetcorn (corn on the cob).

This meat loaf is also delicious if chilled and cut into thin slices, then served as a cold meat with salads, or as a sandwich filling.
The meat loaf can be baked in the oven at 180 °C for 1 hour, although it must then be covered with a lid or aluminium foil.

Dietician's notes
- This dish has a good fibre content due to the lentils added to the mince.
- Sweetcorn (corn on the cob) is a delicious low GI starch to add to any meal, as it also keeps the GL down.

Spaghetti bolognaise

Serves 4

160 g (⅓ packet) spaghetti (durum Wheat)*
500 ml (2 c) boiling water
1 ml (¼ t) salt
5 ml (1 t) olive or canola oil*
1 small onion, peeled and chopped
2 cloves garlic, chopped or 5 ml (1 t) dried garlic flakes
300 g topside mince
10 ml (2 t) beef stock powder
80 ml (generous 5 T) uncooked split lentils* (50 g)
5 ml (1 t) dried sweet basil
5 ml (1 t) dried mixed herbs
1 x 410 g can tomato and onion mix
1 x 65 g or 70 g can tomato paste
15 ml (1 T) Worcester sauce
80 ml red wine (scant ⅓ cup)
250 g (1 punnet) fresh mushrooms, sliced

Nutrients per serving
Glycaemic Index 40 • Carbohydrates 55 g •
Protein 29 g • Fat 9 g • Fibre 8 g • kJ 1 917 •
Glycaemic load 22

ONE SERVING OF SPAGHETTI BOLOGNAISE IS EQUIVALENT
TO 3 PROTEIN + 2 STARCH + VEGETABLES

1 Cook the spaghetti in the boiling water, to which the salt has been added.
2 Heat the oil in a large frying pan and fry the onion and garlic until transparent.
3 Add the mince and beef stock powder; mix well and brown lightly.
4 Add the rest of the ingredients and cook, covered, for about 20 minutes. Add more water if necessary, as the split lentils absorb a lot of liquid. If there is too much sauce, cook uncovered for a few minutes until the liquid has reduced.
5 Serve with spaghetti and vegetables or salad, if desired.
6 Grate a little lower fat cheese on top, if desired.

Add 15 ml (1 T) split lentils per person to any meat casserole or stew. As the lentils cook, they disintegrate and thicken the gravy, so there's no need to use high GI corn-flour or gravy powder as thickening, as the lentils have already done the job.

Dietician's notes
- Please note that the analysis is for the bolognaise sauce and pasta.
- The fat content of the meal will increase if cheese is grated on top, so use lower fat cheese and keep the portion small (½ 'matchbox' per person).
- This bolognaise sauce contains vegetables. Add a fruit for dessert and you don't need to serve a salad with the meal.
- Substituting split lentils for some of the red meat helps to lower the fat content, cholesterol levels and GI of the meal, as well as increasing the fibre content.

See page 120 for Honey mustard dressing, pictured opposite.

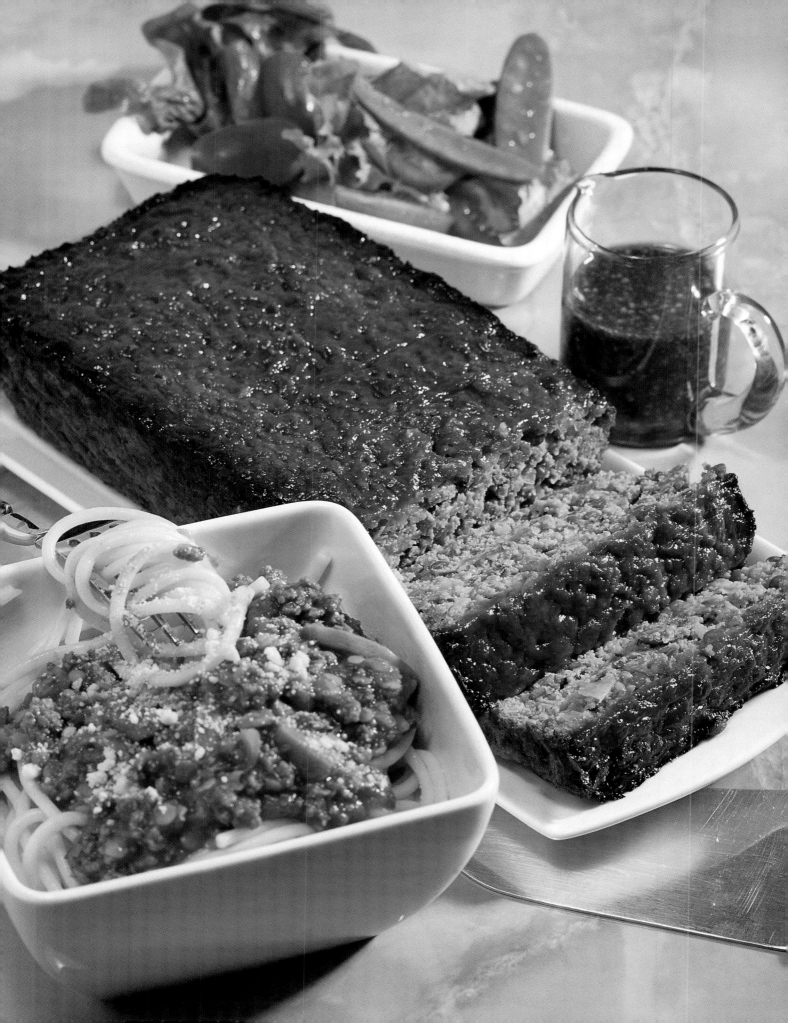

Ostrich bourguignonne

Serves 4

5 ml (1 t) olive oil*
500 g ostrich goulash, cubed
1 medium onion, peeled and chopped
30 ml (2 T) flour
300 ml (1⅕ c) beef stock or 10 ml (2 t) stock powder
    dissolved in 300 ml (1⅕ c) hot water
15 ml (1 T) tomato purée
small bunch fresh herbs or 15 ml (1 T) dried herbs of
    your choice
2 garlic cloves, crushed
90 ml (6 T) red wine
2 ml (½ t) freshly ground black pepper
75 g (about 8) shallots
75 g (about ¼ punet) button mushrooms
5 ml (1 t) butter

1 Preheat the oven to 160 °C, unless you prefer to make this on the stove top.
2 Heat the oil in a frying pan, add half the meat and stir-fry until browned. Transfer to a plate and fry the remaining ostrich and the chopped onion until browned.
3 Return the first batch of ostrich meat to the pan with any meat juices; stir in the flour, then add the stock and the tomato purée. Bring to the boil, and stir until thickened.
4 Add the herbs, garlic, wine and seasoning to the meat and bring to the boil.
5 Cover and cook for 1 hour, or transfer to a casserole dish and bake in the oven for 1 hour, or until the meat is tender.
6 Meanwhile, halve the shallots if large, and wipe and slice the mushrooms. Half an hour before the end of cooking time, fry the shallots in the butter until browned, then add the mushrooms and fry for 2–3 minutes.
7 Stir into the meat and cook for the remaining time.
8 Serve with low GI pasta (boil 160 g uncooked pasta of your choice to serve 4) or low GI rice (boil 185 ml [¾ c] uncooked rice to serve 4) and 2–3 cooked vegetables e.g. Roast vegetables (page 74).

Any other venison meat may be used instead of the ostrich, as venison is equally lean. However, you might have to cook other venison a little longer.

Prepare this casserole at lunchtime and leave it to bake all afternoon in the oven set at a lower temperature, about 140 °C.

Dietician's notes

*   Ostrich meat is almost fat-free. Adding a little butter to this dish is therefore quite acceptable as it is the only saturated fat in the dish, and besides, it adds loads of flavour!
*   Remember that other red meats usually contain saturated fats that increase the risk of heart disease.

Nutrients per serving
(Ostrich and pasta)
Glycaemic Index 40 • Carbohydrates 44 g •
Protein 34 g • Fat 4 g • Fibre 4 g • kJ 1 523 •
Glycaemic load 17

ONE SERVING OF OSTRICH AND PASTA IS EQUIVALENT TO
1½ STARCH + 3 PROTEIN + VEGATABLE

Variation: Venison pie

Serves 4

CRUST
1 egg
125 ml (½ c) fat-free milk*
125 ml (½ c) flour, sifted
15 ml (1 T) baking powder
1 ml (¼ t) salt
65 ml (¼ c) oat bran*, pressed down
15 ml (1 T) 'lite' margarine*, melted

1 Make the filling. Follow steps 2–4 as for Ostrich bourguignonne, but use oats instead of flour, as the crust has a higher GI than pasta. Prepare on top of the stove, not in the oven.
2 Cover and cook the meat in the pot for 30 minutes.
3 Follow steps 6–7 above, cooking uncovered until most of the sauce has evaporated.
4 Preheat the oven to 180 °C. Dish the meat into a slightly greased ovenproof dish.
5 Prepare the crust. Beat the egg and milk together in a mixing bowl.
6 Add the sifted flour, baking powder and salt, as well as the oat bran. Mix thoroughly.
7 Lastly, add the melted margarine and mix through.
8 Spread the crust over the cooked meat and bake for about 30 minutes.
9 Serve with 2 cooked vegetables e.g. Cabbage stir-fry (page 68) and mixed vegetables or salad.

Nutrients per serving
Glycaemic Index 37 • Carbohydrates 28 g •
Protein 33 g • Fat 6 g • Fibre 2 g • kJ 1 337 •
Glycaemic load 10

ONE SERVING IS EQUIVALENT TO
1 STARCH + 3 PROTEIN + VEGETABLE

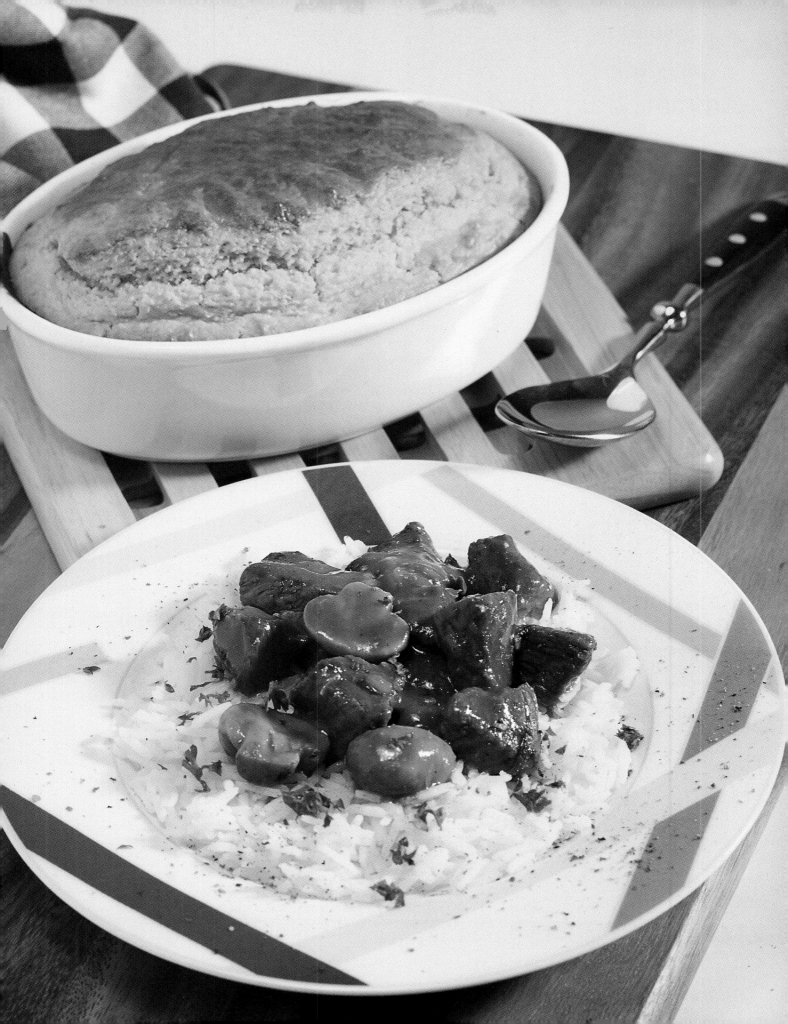

Aromatic fruit salad
Serves 8

15 ml (1 T) sugar (optional)
150 ml (⅗ c) water
1 cinnamon stick or 1 large piece of cassia bark
2 ml (½ t) ginger, crushed
1 whole clove or 1 ml (¼ t) ground cloves
125 ml (½ c) orange juice (1 orange)
500 g (½) honeydew melon (spanspek), peeled,
    seeded and cubed
200 g (1 good-sized wedge) watermelon, cubed
2 ripe guavas or pears
3 ripe nectarines or peaches
150 g (18) strawberries
5 ml (1 t) vanilla essence
300 ml (1⅕ c) fat-free plain yoghurt, for serving
sprigs of mint or rose petals, to decorate

1 First prepare the syrup. Put the sugar (if used), water, cinnamon or cassia, ginger and clove into a saucepan and bring to the boil, stirring to dissolve the sugar. Reduce the temperature and simmer for 2 minutes, then remove from the heat.
2 Add the orange juice and leave to cool and infuse while preparing the fruits.
3 Layer the melon slices in the bottom of a glass bowl.
4 Cut the guavas or pears in half, scoop out the seeds, then peel and slice, dropping each slice into the orange juice to prevent browning. Layer over the melon.
5 Cut the nectarines or peaches into slices, coating with the orange juice to prevent browning as before. Layer over the guavas or pears.
6 Hull and halve the strawberries and layer them over the nectarines or peaches.
7 Strain the syrup, spoon over the sliced fruits and chill for at least 1 hour.
8 Stir the vanilla essence into the yoghurt.
9 Decorate the fruit salad with sprigs of mint or rose petals and serve with a generous dollop of yoghurt 'cream' on each portion.

The spice infusion poured over this fruit salad adds aroma and depth to the flavour. The same spices are added to red wine to make gluhwein (mulled wine).

Dietician's notes

- This is a good example of how one can combine high GI fruits (melons), with low GI fruits to give a low GI dish.
- Omitting the sugar does not lower the GI to any extent. So, even with the sugar, this dessert is suitable for diabetics.
- As this pudding is basically a fruit portion, it can be enjoyed after any main meal in this book.

Nutrients per serving
(fruit salad with 30 ml [2 T] yoghurt)
Glycaemic Index 47 • Carbohydrates 19 g •
Protein 3 g • Fat 0.5 g • Fibre 4 g • kJ 390 •
Glycaemic load 9

ONE SERVING OF FRUIT SALAD AND YOGHURT IS
EQUIVALENT TO 2 FRUIT + A LITTLE DAIRY

Pineapple fluff
Serves 10

250 ml (1 c) rooibos tea
1 x 380 g can low-fat evaporated milk*
1 x 80 g packet pineapple jelly
1 x 410 g can crushed pineapple, drained
2 digestive biscuits, crushed
pineapple pieces and cherries to decorate (optional)

1 Make the rooibos tea, and place the evaporated milk can in the freezer.
2 Add the tea to the jelly powder and stir until completely dissolved.
3 Place in the refrigerator and cool until just starting to set, about 30 minutes.
4 When the jelly is almost set, remove the evaporated milk from the freezer, pour the contents into a large glass bowl, and beat until thick and creamy.
5 Fold the syrupy jelly and crushed pineapple into the beaten milk.
6 Pour the mixture into a serving bowl or dish and refrigerate for at least 1 hour.
7 Sprinkle crushed biscuits over and garnish with pineapple pieces and cherries just before serving.

Any flavour of jelly can be used, as long as it is yellow to match the pineapple. The biscuit topping is optional, but gives the pudding an added crunch.

Dietician's notes

- This pudding is suitable for diabetics, even though it contains ordinary jelly and sweetened canned fruit. Note that we did not use the syrup.
- The low GI evaporated milk lowers the GI of the pudding to acceptable levels.
- As this pudding is low in kilojoules, it can be enjoyed after any one of the main meals in this book.

Nutrients per serving
Glycaemic Index 55 • Carbohydrates 16 g •
Protein 4 g • Fat 2 g • Fibre negl. • kJ 378 •
Glycaemic load 8

ONE SERVING IS EQUIVALENT TO
½ STARCH + ½ DAIRY/MILK

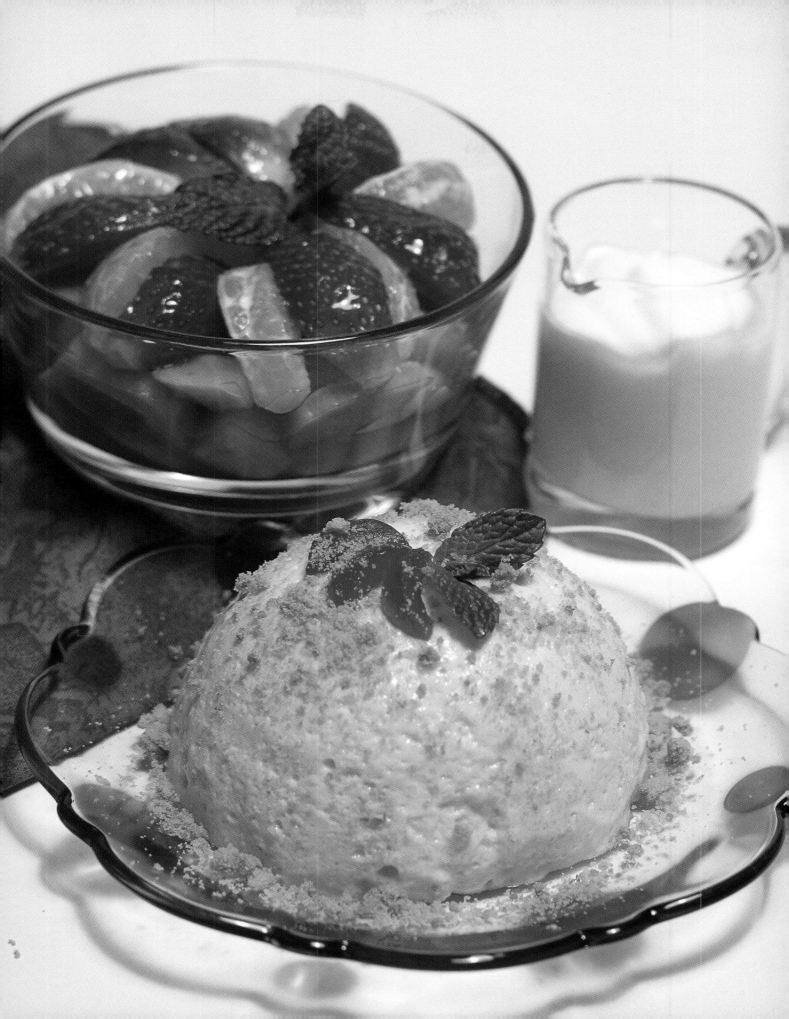

Tipsy tart
Serves 12

125 g dates, chopped
100 ml (⅖ c) boiling water
10 ml (2 t) bicarbonate of soda
250 ml (1 c) small white (or butter) beans*, mashed
1 large apple or 2 small apples, grated
15 ml (1 T) canola or olive oil
200 ml (⅘ c) soft brown sugar
2 eggs, beaten
5 ml (1 t) vanilla essence
125 ml (½ c) flour
5 ml (1 t) baking powder
pinch of salt
125 ml (½ c) oat bran*, pressed down
125 ml (½ c) high-fibre cereal*, crushed
12 pecan nut halves, chopped
SAUCE
250 ml (1 c) peach and orange juice mix*
5 ml (1 t) vanilla essence
65 ml (¼ c) brandy

Nutrients per serving

Glycaemic Index 58 • Carbohydrates 31 g •
Protein 4 g • Fat 4 g • Fibre 4 g • kJ 758 •
Glycaemic load 18

ONE SERVING (WITHOUT THE EVAPORATED MILK) IS
EQUIVALENT TO 2 STARCH + 1 FAT

---

1 Preheat the oven to 180 °C.
2 Pour the boiling water over the dates. Allow to stand for a while, so that the dates can soften, and then mash them. Add the bicarbonate of soda and stir until the mixture foams.
3 Mix the beans and apple into the date mixture and leave to cool.
4 Stir in the oil and sugar, then the beaten eggs and vanilla essence.
5 Sift the flour, baking powder and salt together, and gradually add all the dry ingredients to the mixture.
6 Pour into a lightly greased pie dish and bake for 50 minutes. Slice while hot.
7 SAUCE: Boil all the ingredients together for 5 minutes and pour over the hot tart.
8 Serve with chilled, beaten, low-fat ('lite') evaporated milk.

250 ml (1 c) small white beans, cooked, is equivalent to 1 x 410 g can of small white beans, drained.

Dietician's notes

- When adding mashed beans to your own recipes, 250 ml (1 c) is about as much as you will be able to add per recipe. Remember to add 5 ml (1 t) baking powder to ensure a light texture, and reduce the liquid by about one-third.
- This is a deliciously moist tart. It can be eaten on its own, or served with whipped, chilled lower fat evaporated milk or low-fat ice cream.
- This is an ideal way to incorporate beans into your family's diet. The Tipsy tart is delicious, and one cannot taste the beans at all!
- Please note that, because this pudding contains 2 starches, you should omit the starch from the meal with which you're serving it.
- Note the fibre content, considering that puddings do not usually contain fibre.

Caramelised yoghurt and fruit
Serves 4

400–500 g (2 punnets) strawberries or other berries
2 x 175 ml tubs yoghurt* (plain, low-fat or fat-free) or 350 ml (1 ⅖ c) plain yoghurt
45 ml (3 T) soft brown sugar

Nutrients per serving

Glycaemic Index 35 • Carbohydrates 21 g •
Protein 5 g • Fat 2 g • Fibre 3 g • kJ 525 •
Glycaemic load 7

ONE SERVING IS EQUIVALENT TO
½ DAIRY + 1 FRUIT

---

1 Place the berries in a serving dish and spoon the yoghurt over the fruit.
2 Sprinkle the sugar on top and leave in the fridge for a few hours or overnight so that the sugar can 'caramelise'.

Dietician's notes

- Two medium mangoes may be used instead of the berries, but if you use 500 g mango in place of the berries, the GI rises to 47 and the GL to 16, as mangoes are higher in carbohydrate and have a higher GI than berries.
- This dessert is a good example of how very low GI plain yoghurt can be used to offset higher GI sugar (and mangoes, if used) and therefore this dish is completely safe for diabetics, in spite of the presence of the sugar.
- For a creamier taste, use double cream yoghurt (6.6 g fat per 100 g) or low-fat cream (12.3 g fat per 100 g). Although this is much higher in fat (6–11 g fat per portion) than when low-fat yoghurt is used (2 g fat per portion), it is still much lower in fat than regular cream, which contains 37–50 g fat per 100 g, and yields 32–44 g fat per portion of this dessert!
- Remember that cream is a saturated fat source, and not the healthiest choice.

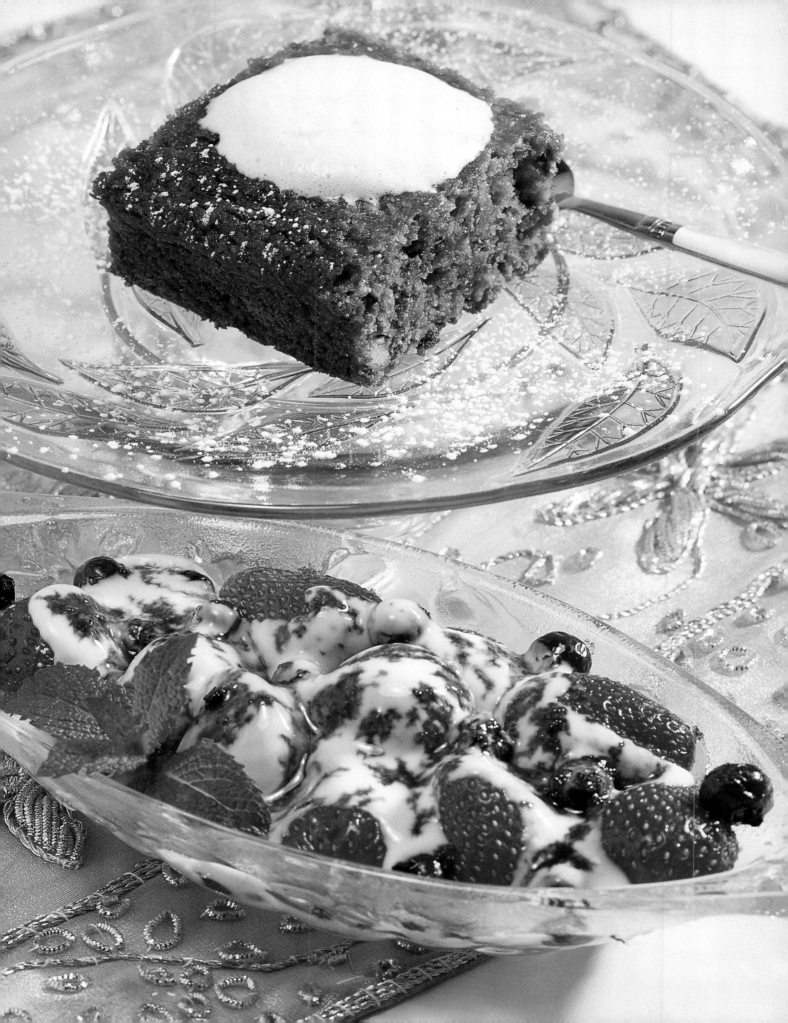

Forest berry pudding

Serves 6

250 g low-fat cottage cheese*
80 ml (scant ⅓ c) sugar
1 x 175 ml tub low-fat berry yoghurt*
2 eggs, separated
15 ml (1 T) gelatine powder
60 ml (4 T) cold water
5 ml (1 t) vanilla essence
pinch of salt
1 x 410 g can berries in natural juice
10 ml (2 t) cornflour

1 Whisk the cottage cheese, sugar, yoghurt and egg yolks until smooth.
2 Soften the gelatine in the cold water and dissolve slowly over low heat, or microwave on high for 10 seconds, stir, and microwave again for 10 seconds on high to dissolve the gelatine completely.
3 Gradually beat the gelatine into the cheese mixture. Stir in the vanilla essence.
4 Whisk the egg whites and salt until stiff (be sure to use clean beaters), then fold the egg whites into the cottage cheese mixture, using a metal spoon.
5 Pour into a clean bowl and refrigerate for 45 minutes, or until set firmly.
6 When the pudding is set, drain the fruit (reserve the juice) and mash lightly if necessary.
7 Stir the cornflour into the reserved juice until smooth. Heat in a saucepan until the mixture thickens and is transparent. Leave to cool.
8 Meanwhile, arrange the fruit on top of the pudding.
9 When the juice is cool to the touch, spoon the cooled thickened juice evenly over the fruit until all the fruit is just covered. Discard any excess.
10 Return to fridge until set completely.

Strawberry, raspberry or mixed berry yoghurt can be used. Make sure it is low fat. Any canned or fresh or frozen berries can be used for the topping.

Dietician's notes

- Although high GI cornflour is used to thicken the fruit juice, the GI of the pudding is low, as all the other low GI ingredients offset the high GI cornflour.
- Using berries in regular syrup is quite acceptable, even for those with diabetes, when combined with a diary product (yoghurt or milk), as the low GI dairy offsets the higher GI sugar syrup.

Nutrients per serving
Glycaemic Index 43 • Carbohydrates 25 g •
Protein 10 g • Fat 2 g • Fibre 1 g • kJ 677 •
Glycaemic load 11

ONE SERVING OF PUDDING IS EQUIVALENT TO
1 STARCH + ½ FRUIT + 1 DAIRY

Spicy baked pudding

Serves 8

375 ml (1½ c) fat-free milk*, warmed
125 ml (½ c) high-fibre cereal*
3 large eggs
125 ml (½ c) soft brown sugar
400 g (2 medium) sweet potatoes, peeled and grated
2 ml (½ t) salt
2 ml (½ t) ground cinnamon
1 ml (¼ t) grated nutmeg
1 ml (¼ t) ground ginger
1 ml (¼ t) ground cloves
125 ml (½ c) sultanas
12 walnut or pecan nut halves (optional)

1 Preheat the oven to 180 °C and lightly grease a medium-sized ovenproof dish.
2 Pour the milk over the cereal and set aside.
3 Beat the eggs, gradually adding the brown sugar.
4 Add the sweet potato to the egg mixture.
5 Add the cereal and milk, salt, spices and sultanas, and mix well.
6 Pour into the prepared dish, and even out the raw ingredients within the mix.
7 Place the walnuts or pecan nuts decoratively on top of the pudding.
8 Bake for about 1 hour, or until firm to the touch.

The finer you grate the sweet potato, the better the flavours will combine and give a spicier, richer pudding.

Beating the sugar gradually into the eggs improves the volume and texture.

Dietician's notes

- The original recipe contained honey. We had to use soft brown sugar instead of honey, because honey is very dense in carbohydrates and kilojoules, resulting in double the GL. If you would prefer to use honey, use only 65 ml (¼ c).
- Remember to omit the starch in your main course if you are having this pudding at the same meal.

Nutrients per serving
Glycaemic Index 54 • Carbohydrates 32 g •
Protein 6 g • Fat 4 g • Fibre 4 g • kJ 788 •
Glycaemic load 17

ONE SERVING OF PUDDING IS EQUIVALENT TO
2 STARCH + 1 DAIRY/PROTEIN

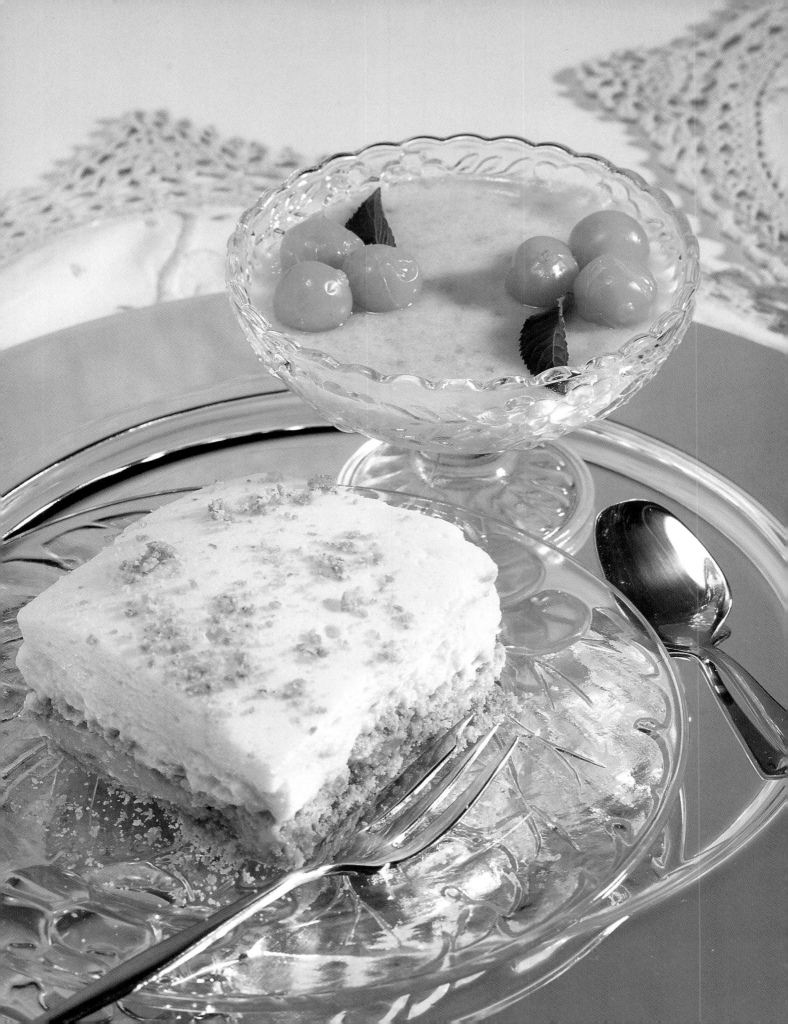

Melktert (Milk tart)

Serves 12

Makes 2 small tarts or 1 large tart

BASE

125 ml (½ c) high-fibre cereal*
75–80 ml (5 T or ⅓ c) warm skimmed milk*
250 ml (1 c) cake flour
2 ml (½ t) salt
2 ml (½ t) baking powder
75–80 ml (5 T or scant ⅓ c) soft brown sugar
1 egg, beaten
20 ml (4 t) canola or olive oil

FILLING

250 ml (1 c) skimmed milk*
80 ml (scant ⅓ c) soft brown sugar
45 ml (3 T) cake flour
2 ml (½ t) salt
45 ml (3 T) water
250 ml (1 c) fat-free plain yoghurt*
5 ml (1 t) vanilla essence
15 ml (1 T) 'lite' margarine*
2 eggs, lightly beaten
5 ml (1 t) ground cinnamon

1 Make the base. Measure out the cereal and pour the warm milk over it. Leave to stand until the cereal is soft and the milk has been absorbed.
2 Sift the flour, salt and baking powder into a mixing bowl.
3 Mash the now soft high-fibre cereal, and add to the flour mixture, together with the sugar, beaten egg and the oil.
4 With a wooden spoon, gently mix to form a dough.
5 Spoon half the dough into each of 2 lightly greased small pie dishes (20 cm in diameter), and smooth into a thin layer with the back of a tablespoon, or using your fingers.
6 Bake for 10–12 minutes at 180 °C. While the bases are baking, make the filling.
7 Pour the milk into a 1 litre (4 c) jug and microwave on high for 2 minutes, or pour the milk into a saucepan and heat until nearly boiling.
8 Meanwhile, make a smooth paste from the sugar, flour, salt and water in a small bowl.
9 Pour some of the hot milk onto the flour and sugar paste and stir well.
10 Then pour the sugar and flour mixture back into the rest of the hot milk and stir.
11 Microwave on high for 1 minute. Stir, and microwave on high for another 2–3 minutes, 30 seconds at a time, stirring after each 30 seconds of heating, or until the custard is smooth and thick.
12 Alternatively, bring to the boil on the stove top, stirring, until thick and smooth.
13 Leave to cool for 10 minutes, then stir in the yoghurt.
14 Stir in the vanilla essence, margarine and eggs.
15 Pour into the baked pastry shells, sprinkle with the ground cinnamon, and bake at 250 °C for 10 minutes.
16 Turn the heat down to 180 °C and bake for a further 15 minutes.
17 Leave to cool before serving.

The yoghurt gives this Melktert a slightly sour tang. If you prefer not to use yoghurt, simply use skimmed milk in its place, but the filling will then be less firm.
The cinnamon gives the Melktert its typical flavour.
This pastry can be successfully used as a base for any other kind of sweet tart.
Using a wire whisk to stir the custard filling ensures a smooth, lump-free custard.

Dietician's notes

- We used half yoghurt and half skimmed milk to give a good texture, as we had to use this to lower the effect of the high GI flour needed for thickening the filling.
- Remember to omit at least one starch at your meal if you are having Melktert for pudding.
- A Glycaemic load of 15 is quite high for an 'extra' at a meal. Make sure the meal you eat before this pudding contains lots of vegetables.

Nutrients per slice (1/12 large tart)
Glycaemic Index 59 • Carbohydrates 22 g •
Protein 5 g • Fat 4 g • Fibre 1 g • kJ 593 •
Glycaemic load 15

ONE SMALL SLICE IS EQUIVALENT TO
1½ STARCH + ½ DAIRY

Health bread

Makes 20 slices

250 ml (1 c) cake flour
2 ml (½ t) salt
5 ml (1 t) baking powder
250 ml (1 c) whole-wheat flour, e.g. Nutty Wheat
250 ml (1 c) high-fibre cereal*
250 ml (1 c) lower GI oats*
125 ml (½ c) sultanas
60 ml (4 T) sunflower seeds
5 ml (1 t) bicarbonate of soda
500 ml (2 c) low-fat plain or fruit yoghurt*

1   Preheat the oven to 180 °C.
2   Sift the cake flour, salt and baking powder into a bowl.
3   Stir in the whole-wheat flour, the cereal, oats, sultanas and sunflower seeds.
4   Add the bicarbonate of soda to the yoghurt and set aside for a couple of minutes or until it foams lightly. Stir into the dry ingredients.
5   Spoon into a 30 cm long bread pan that has been sprayed with nonstick spray.
6   Bake for about 1 hour, or until the loaf recedes from the sides of the pan.
7   Tip the loaf out of the pan and leave to cool before slicing.

Remember, this bread has to bake for an hour, so plan ahead!
This bread can also be made in a cast iron pot over an open fire.

Dietician's notes

•   This delicious, easy to make, lower GI alternative to ordinary, high GI bread, can be eaten at breakfast, with a light meal or at a braai.
•   Note that seeds are high in fat – albeit a beneficial fat – and for this reason we have used only 60 ml (4 T).
•   Please note that the analysis is for the bread made with plain yoghurt. If sweetened fruit yoghurt is used, the GI will be lowered slightly to 56, but the GL goes up to 12, so use whichever you prefer.

Nutrients per slice

Glycaemic Index 57 • Carbohydrates 18 g •
Protein 4 g • Fat 2 g • Fibre 3 g • kJ 478 •
Glycaemic load 10

ONE SLICE IS EQUIVALENT TO
1 STARCH + ½ FAT

Mealie bread

Makes 18 slices

500 ml (2 c) self-raising flour
2 ml (½ t) salt
5 ml (1 t) mustard powder
250 ml (1 c) oat bran*
250 ml (1 c) whole-wheat ProNutro*
60 ml (4 T) soft 'lite' margarine*, melted
1 egg
125 ml (½ c) low-fat or fat-free milk*, or low-fat buttermilk*, or low-fat plain yoghurt*
1 x 410 g can creamstyle sweetcorn

1   Preheat the oven to 180 °C.
2   Sift self-raising flour, salt and mustard powder together into a large bowl.
3   Add the oat bran and ProNutro, and lift up dry ingredients a few times with a spoon to incorporate air.
4   Melt the margarine in the microwave on high for 30 seconds. Add the egg and beat well with a fork. Add the milk or buttermilk or yoghurt. Mix thoroughly.
5   Add the wet ingredients (including the sweetcorn) to the dry ingredients. Mix gently to cover all the dry ingredients with the wet ingredients. Don't overmix, as this improves digestibility and raises the GI.
6   Spoon the sticky dough into a 30 cm long bread pan that has been sprayed with nonstick spray, and smooth the top of the bread with the back of a metal spoon.
7   Bake for about 1½ hours.
8   Tip the baked bread out of the loaf pan and leave it on a wire cooling rack to cool down before cutting into 18 slices.

This bread must either be eaten fresh, or frozen (sliced) for later use. When required, simply pop a frozen slice of mealie bread into the toaster to defrost.
Use 500 ml [2 c] flour and 10 ml [2 t] baking powder instead of the 500 ml self-raising flour.

Dietician's notes

•   This delicious, lower GI bread can be enjoyed as the starch at a braai or with a light meal, together with low-fat protein and salad.

See page 120 for Hummus recipe (pictured next to Health bread).
See page 121 for Aubergine pâté recipe (pictured next to Mealie bread).

Nutrients per slice

Glycaemic Index 62 • Carbohydrates 19 g •
Protein 4 g • Fat 3 g • Fibre 3 g • kJ 528 •
Glycaemic load 12

ONE SLICE IS EQUIVALENT TO
1½ STARCH + ½ FAT

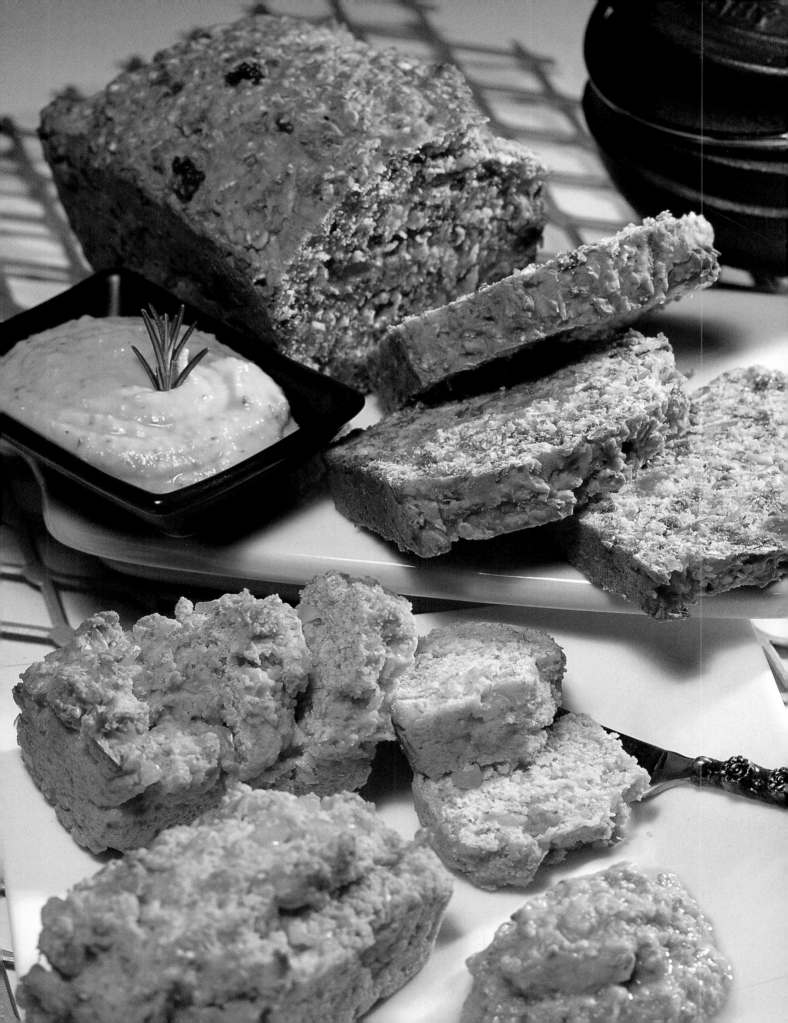

Onion bread

Makes 16 slices

750 ml (3 c) self-raising flour
250 ml (1 c) oat bran*
5 ml (1 t) baking powder
1x 100 g packet flavoured soya mince* (tomato and
    onion, or any other flavour)
1 fresh apple, grated
½ onion, peeled and chopped finely
500 ml (2 c) fat-free plain yoghurt*
150 ml (⅗ c) water
½ onion, peeled and sliced into rings

1   Preheat the oven to 180 °C.
2   Sift the flour into a large bowl; add the oat bran and baking powder and mix.
3   Add the uncooked soya mince, and lift up a few times to incorporate air.
4   Add the grated apple and chopped onion, and mix in gently.
5   Add the yoghurt and water, and stir just enough to combine, adding extra water if necessary.
6   Spoon into a greased 30 cm long loaf pan. Press the onion rings into the top.
7   Bake for 2 hours. Test the loaf by inserting a clean knife or skewer into the centre. If it comes out clean, the bread is done. If not, bake for another 10 minutes.
8   Stand on a rack to cool before slicing.

This deliciously moist bread is ideal for meals enjoyed al fresco. It only keeps for a day, so slice and freeze the rest, defrosting each slice in a toaster, as needed. Instead of self-raising flour, use 5 ml (1 t) baking powder per 250 ml (1 c) of flour.

Dietician's notes

*   This tasty loaf is dense and heavy, because it is a low GI bread.
*   We used the soya (mince), a legume, to lower the GI of this bread.
*   Soya can be used very effectively to lower the GI of any meal. For example, use 1 x 100 g packet of soya mince with 500 g lean mince when making mince dishes to lower the GI and the fat content of that meal.

Nutrients per slice

Glycaemic Index 56 • Carbohydrates 26 g •
Protein 6 g • Fat 1 g • Fibre 3 g • kJ 594 •
Glycaemic load 15

ONE SLICE IS EQUIVALENT TO
1½ STARCH + ½ PROTEIN/DAIRY

Gingerbread

Makes 14 slices

80–90 ml (scant ⅓ c to 6 T) soft 'lite' margarine*
250 ml (1 c) wheat rice* (stampkoring or pearled
    wheat), cooked
125 ml (½ c) soft brown sugar
250 ml (1 c) oat bran*
60 ml (4 T) raw honey
250 ml (1 c) cake flour
125 ml (½ c) skimmed milk*
10 ml (2 t) instant coffee powder
1 egg
5 ml (1 t) ground ginger
2 ml (½ t) salt
5 ml (1 t) bicarbonate of soda
5 ml (1 t) baking powder

1   Preheat the oven to 180 °C.
2   Place the margarine in a mixing bowl and soften it, using a wooden spoon.
3   Add the cooked wheat rice, sugar, oat bran and honey. Sift the flour and mix in.
4   Heat the milk and dissolve the coffee powder in it. Beat the egg into the milk and coffee mixture. Add to the dry ingredients and mix well.
5   Add the ginger, salt, bicarbonate of soda and baking powder. Mix in thoroughly.
6   Pour the batter into a lightly greased 25 cm x 10 cm loaf pan.
7   Bake for 1 hour. Remove from the oven and cool.

This cake sinks slightly in the middle and tastes best if stored in an airtight container for 24 hours before eating, so that the ginger flavour has time to develop. The cooked wheat rice goes hard and tastes like nuts in the cake.

It is important to add the bicarbonate of soda and baking powder at the end, after the hot milk, to ensure that the cake will rise well.

Dietician's notes

*   This bread will become crumbly if stored for more than 2–3 days. For a less crumbly bread, use 312 ml (1¼ c) cake flour and 187 ml (¾ c) oat bran.
*   It is important to use raw honey, as other honey and syrups have a higher GI.
*   The gingerbread slices can be 'buttered' with a little fat-free cottage cheese sweetened with 10 ml (2 t) jam per 125 g fat-free cottage cheese*.
*   It is interesting to note that the GI of Mealie bread (a savoury bread) is similar to the GI of this Gingerbread (a cake). (See page 96 for the Mealie bread recipe.)

Nutrients per slice

Glycaemic Index 60 • Carbohydrates 23 g •
Protein 3 g • Fat 4 g • Fibre 2 g • kJ 575 •
Glycaemic load 14

ONE SLICE IS EQUIVALENT TO
1½ STARCH + 1 FAT

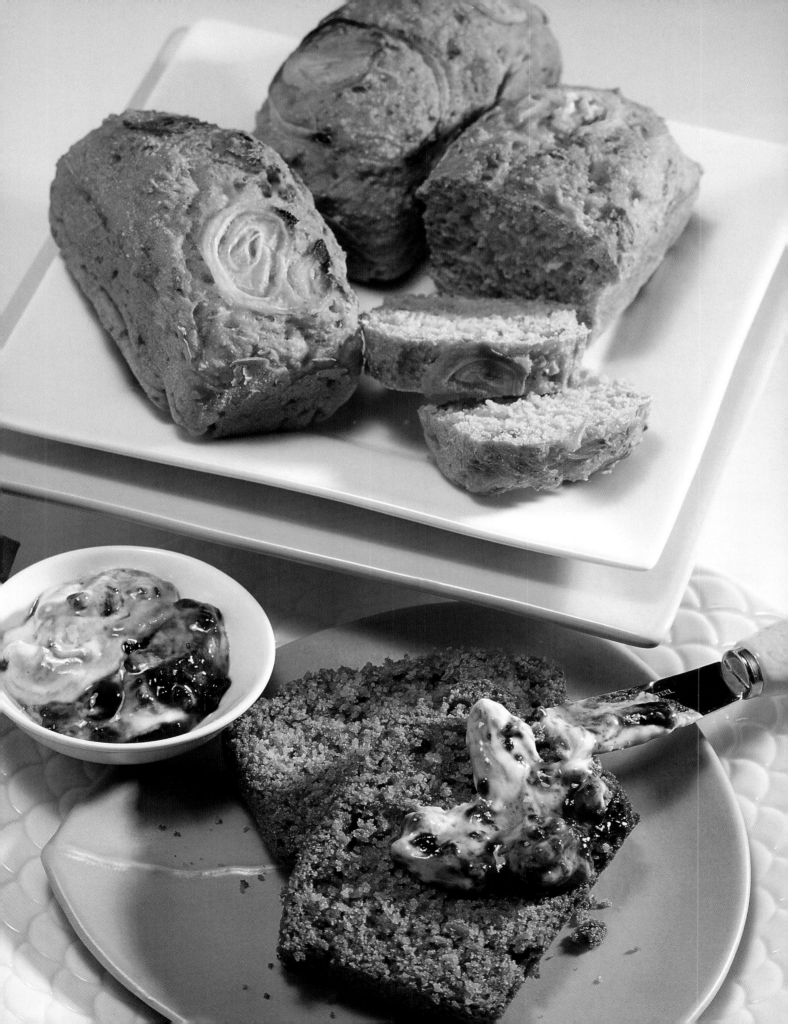

Banana bread

Makes 14 slices

2 bananas
30 ml (2 T) lemon juice
1 small apple, grated
100 ml (⅖ c) skimmed (fat-free) milk*
250 ml (1 c) high-fibre cereal*
10 ml (2 t) canola or macadamia oil*
125 ml (½ c) soft brown sugar
1 egg
250 ml (1 c) cake flour
10 ml (2 t) baking powder
2 ml (½ t) salt
5 ml (1 t) vanilla essence

1   Preheat the oven to 180 °C while you prepare the batter.
2   Peel the bananas and mash the flesh with the lemon juice.
3   Mix the grated apple into the mashed banana. Set aside.
4   Heat the milk and pour it over the high-fibre cereal. Stir and leave to soften.
5   Cream the oil, sugar and egg until smooth, but not for longer than 1 minute.
6   Sift together the flour, baking powder and salt in a separate mixing bowl.
7   Combine the sifted dry ingredients, the soaked cereal, and the apple and banana, and stir well, using a wooden spoon.
8   Add the vanilla essence and stir in.
9   Spoon into a greased loaf pan, about 30 cm long, and level the surface of the bread mixture.
10 Bake for 1 hour.
11 Switch off the oven and leave the cake in the oven for another 10 minutes.
12 Remove the cake from the oven; gently remove it from the baking pan, and cool on a wire rack.

This cake needs to bake for a longer time at a lower heat because of the high fruit content; cakes containing fruit tend to burn easily.

Microwaving the cake gives a much lighter texture, although the colour is no longer golden brown. See below for microwave method.

Dietician's note

• One slice of this cake contains only 1 g of fat. This means it would be acceptable to spread a little margarine (or butter) over, if desired.

Microwave method

1   Line the base of a microwave loaf pan with a paper towel cut to size.
2   Spray lightly with nonstick oil.
3   Spoon the batter into the loaf pan, filling it not more than half way. Level the batter.
4   Microwave on high for 6 minutes.
5   Insert a toothpick near the centre (but not in the centre); if it comes out clean, the cake is ready to be removed from the microwave oven.
6   If not, continue microwaving, for 30 seconds at a time, until a toothpick inserted into the centre to test for doneness, comes out clean.
7   Place the cake on a solid surface and leave it to stand for 6 minutes so that the base can continue to cook, before removing it from the loaf pan.
8   Run a knife around all 4 sides to loosen the cake. Invert it onto a cooling rack.
9   Remove (peel away) the paper towel.

Nutrients per slice

Glycaemic Index 59 • Carbohydrates 19 g •
Protein 3 g • Fat 1 g • Fibre 3 g • kJ 424 •
Glycaemic load 11

ONE SLICE IS EQUIVALENT TO
1½ STARCH

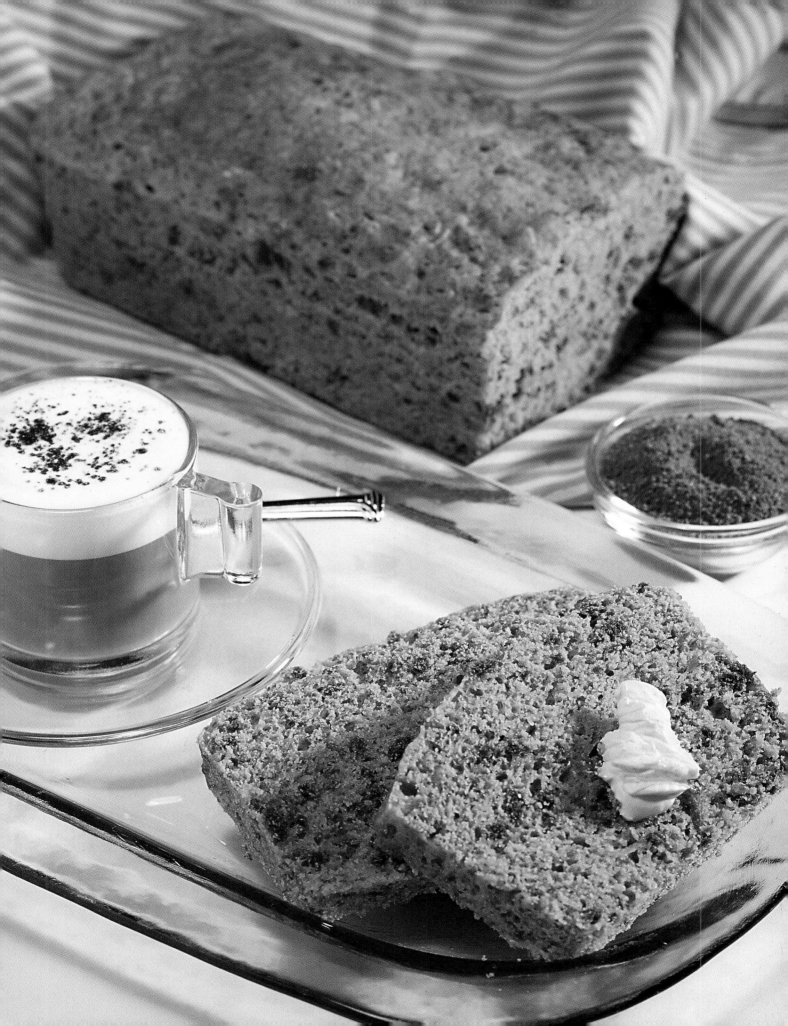

Traditional German baked cheesecake

Makes 16 slices

BASE

125 ml (½ c) high-fibre bran cereal*
60 ml (4 T) warm skimmed milk*
250 ml (1 c) cake flour
2 ml (½ t) salt
2 ml (½ t) baking powder
85 ml (⅓ c) soft brown sugar
1 egg, beaten
30 ml (2 T) canola or macadamia oil*

FILLING

750–800 g fat-free cottage cheese* (4 x 200 g tubs
    or 3 x 250 g tubs)
3 eggs, separated
175 ml (generous ⅔ c) sugar
15 ml (1 T) cornflour
2 ml (½ t) vanilla essence
15 ml (1 T) lemon juice
10 ml (2 t) grated lemon zest
75 g (½ c) sultanas

1   First make the base. Measure out the high-fibre cereal and pour the warm milk over it. Set aside.
2   Sift the flour, salt and baking powder into a mixing bowl.
3   Add the sugar to the dry ingredients and stir until all the sugar crystals are separate and coated with the dry ingredients.
4   Mash the now soft high-fibre cereal and add it to the flour mixture, together with the beaten egg and the oil.
5   Using a wooden spoon, mix gently to form a dough.
6   Spoon the dough into a spring-form cake tin and smooth into a thin layer, using the back of a tablespoon or your fingers.
7   Refrigerate for 10 minutes.
8   Preheat the oven to 180 °C.
9   Make the filling. Mix the cottage cheese in a bowl with the egg yolks and sugar.
10 Sift the cornflour over and fold it in.
11 Add the vanilla essence, lemon juice and zest.
12 Mix well until blended, then stir in the sultanas.
13 Whisk the egg whites and fold them in.
14 Pour into the pastry-lined baking tin and bake for 70 minutes, or until golden.
15 Switch the oven off and leave the cheesecake in the warm oven for 30 minutes, to stop the filling from wrinkling.
16 Cool completely, before removing from the baking pan.

Pastry is notoriously difficult to make. This recipe follows a different method as we have had to substitute as much high-fibre bran cereal for the high GI flour as possible. You will, however, be pleasantly surprised at how easy it is to make, and how good it tastes.

For a creamier flavour to the filling, replace 1 tub of fat-free cottage cheese with 1 tub low-fat cream cheese or 3–4 tubs of low-fat cottage cheese. Remember, however, that the fat content of the cheesecake will then be higher (6–8 g fat per portion), which means you should compensate for this extra fat at the next meal by omitting one fat from the meal, as well as the starch.

Dietician's notes

*   Cheesecake fillings are usually made using at least half cream and half cream cheese, and the cakes thus have a very high fat content. Using fat-free cottage cheese effectively lowers the fat content … so go ahead, enjoy this delicious and nutritious version of the high-fat favourite.
*   Please note that this cake should be cut into 16 slices.
*   This cheesecake can be eaten as a pudding or as a snack. Remember, however, to omit at least one of the starches at one of your meals.

Nutrients per slice
Glycaemic Index 60 • Carbohydrates 25 g •
Protein 9 g • Fat 4 g • Fibre 1 g • kJ 714 •
Glycaemic load 15

ONE SLICE IS EQUIVALENT TO
1 STARCH + 1 DAIRY/MILK

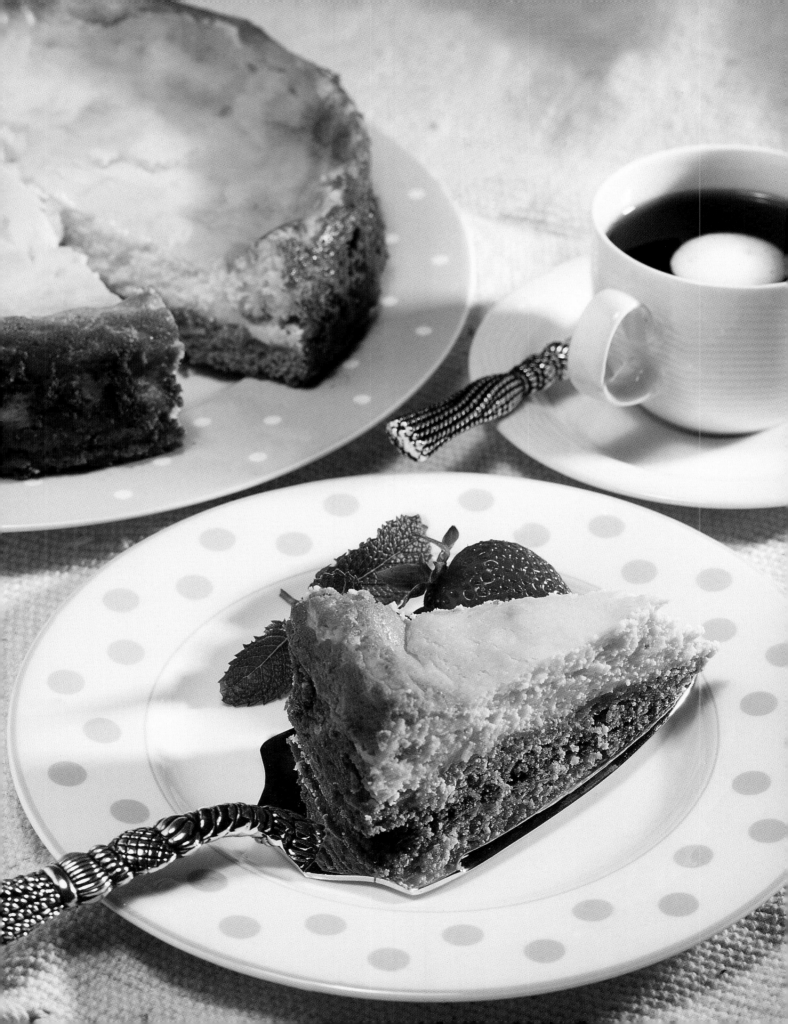

Christmas fruit cake

Makes 20 portions

250 ml (1 c) water
125 ml (½ c) fat-free milk*
125 ml (½ c) soft 'lite' margarine*
125 ml (½ c) sultanas
35 (½ x 250 g packet) dried apricot halves, roughly chopped
12 (½ x 250 g packet) dried prunes
10 (½ x 250 g packet) dried peach halves, roughly chopped
30 ml (2 T) currants
125 ml (½ c) white sugar
5 ml (1 t) bicarbonate of soda
1 ml (¼ t) salt
10 pecan nut halves, chopped
190 ml (¾ c) cake flour
5 ml (1 t) bicarbonate of soda
5 ml (1 t) baking powder
85 ml (⅓ c) oat bran*
250 ml (1 c) whole-wheat ProNutro*
1 apple, peeled and very finely grated
1 egg
2 ml (½ t) almond essence
1 egg white, beaten

1 Place the water, milk, margarine, fruit, sugar, 5 ml (1 t) bicarbonate of soda, the salt and nuts in a large saucepan. Simmer over low heat for 20 minutes.
2 Remove from the heat, pour into a bowl and allow to cool completely.
3 Remove the pips from the prunes. Preheat the oven to 160 °C.
4 Sift together the flour, 5 ml (1 t) bicarbonate of soda, and the baking powder over the cooled fruits in the bowl.
5 Add the oat bran, the whole-wheat ProNutro and the grated apple.
6 Mix gently with a wooden spoon.
7 Beat the egg and almond essence together, and add to the batter.
8 Whisk the egg white and fold it into the mixture.
9 Spoon the batter into a nonstick baking pan (a 30 cm long loaf pan or 15 cm square or round pan), which has been sprayed with nonstick spray.
10 Bake for 2 hours, or until a knife or skewer inserted into the centre comes out clean.
11 Allow to cool completely, then sprinkle with a little brandy (optional).
12 Store in an airtight container, or cover with foil and store for 2 days in the fridge before eating.

This fruit cake has a high fruit content, which makes it very moist, so it is best stored in the fridge, otherwise it could become mouldy.
Chilled fruit cake is rather delicious … try it!

Microwave method

1 Place the fruit and the other ingredients listed in step 1 above into a glass bowl and microwave on medium/low for 5–6 minutes.
2 Follow the recipe above from step 2–8.
3 Line a microwave pan with a paper towel, and spray with nonstick spray.
4 Spoon the batter into the pan and microwave on medium for 18–20 minutes. The cake is done when the top is no longer moist.
5 Remove from the microwave pan and carefully peel off the paper.
6 Allow to cool completely, then sprinkle with a little brandy (optional).
7 Store in an airtight container or cover with foil and store for 2 days in the fridge before eating.

Dietician's notes

- Note the low GI, low GL and low-fat content of this cake. Remember to cut it into 20 pieces.
- The original GI of the fruit cake was 65. By replacing some of the flour with whole-wheat ProNutro and oat bran, as well as making a few other alterations, we succeeded in lowering the GI of the cake to less than 50!
- Very few cakes contain as much fibre and as little fat per portion as this fruit cake.
- Christmas cakes usually contain more flour and more fat in the form of suet, but they are still lower GI and lower fat than most other cakes.

Nutrients per piece of cake
Glycaemic Index 49 • Carbohydrates 26 g • Protein 3 g • Fat 4 g • Fibre 3 g • kJ 673 • Glycaemic load 13

ONE PIECE OF CAKE IS EQUIVALENT TO
1 STARCH + 1 FRUIT + 1 FAT

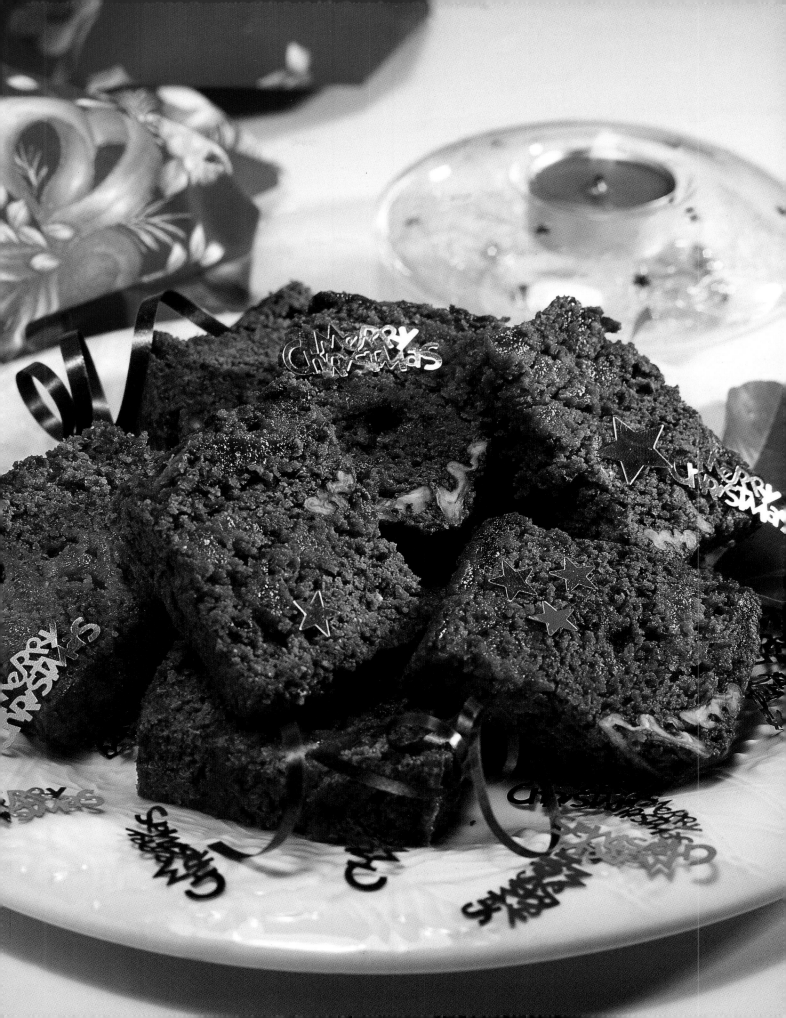

Chocolate cake

Makes 20 slices

200 g (1 medium) sweet potato, peeled and cubed
5 (1 t) bicarbonate of soda
60 ml (4 T) canola or macadamia oil*
125 ml (½ c) boiling water
100 ml (⅖ c) cocoa powder
375 ml (1½ c) cake flour
1 ml (¼ t) salt
20 ml (4 t) baking powder
125 ml (½ c) oatbran*
2 eggs
2 egg whites
190 ml (¾ c) castor sugar or 250 ml (1c) Sugalite
5 ml (1 t) vanilla essence
125 ml (½ c) low-fat buttermilk* or plain yoghurt*
1 large apple, peeled and grated
30 ml (2 T) low GI apricot jam*
CHOCOLATE ICING
60 ml (4 T) icing sugar or 90 ml (6 T) Sugalite
25 ml (5 t) cocoa powder
200–250 g fat-free or low-fat cottage cheese*
5 ml (1 t) rum essence

1 Preheat the oven to 180 ˚C.
2 Boil the sweet potato until tender; drain and mash. Add the bicarbonate of soda to the warm, mashed sweet potato; stir in lightly and leave to 'foam'.
3 Place the oil and boiling water in a saucepan on the stove and sift in the cocoa powder. Stir until dissolved and bring to the boil. Place in the fridge to cool.
4 In another bowl, sift the flour, salt and baking powder. Add the oat bran and lift up a few times with a spoon to incorporate air.
5 Beat the eggs and egg whites for 2 minutes in a large mixing bowl, using electric beaters. Add the castor sugar in 2 batches, beating for 1 minute after each addition.
6 Remove the cocoa and oil mixture from the fridge and stir in the vanilla essence, the yoghurt or buttermilk, and the apple and the sweet potato mixture.
7 Add a third of this mixture to the egg mixture, alternating with the flour mixture. Fold in lightly after each addition until well blended. Ensure that the cocoa mixture does not sink to the bottom.
8 Pour the batter into 2 cake tins that have been sprayed with nonstick spray. Spread the batter out towards the sides, so that the cake does not rise too high in the centre during baking.
9 Bake for 30–40 minutes, or until a toothpick inserted into the centre comes out clean. Remove from the oven and leave to cool in the tin. Loosen the sides with a knife before removing the cake from the tin.
10 Sift the icing sugar and cocoa powder into the cottage cheese and add the rum essence. Mix thoroughly, but do not overmix.
11 Sandwich the 2 cake layers together with the apricot jam, and spread the icing over the top of the cake.

This is an ideal recipe in which to use a polydextrose-based product, such as Sugalite, to lower the GI and improve the texture of the cake. Use 250 ml (1 c) Sugalite instead of the sugar in the cake recipe and 90 ml (6 T) Sugalite instead of the icing sugar in the icing. Each slice will now have a lower GI (below 55), slightly less kilojoules, but still 4 g fat per slice. See pages 13–14 for a discussion of polydextrose and lactitol, the ingredients in Sugalite.

Do not eat more than 1 slice of cake if you are using Sugalite, as 1 slice already contains 13 g of Sugalite; an intake of 20 g or more of Sugalite may cause flatulence, cramping and/or diarrhoea.

Sugalite is not suitable for those suffering from a spastic colon or Irritable Bowel Syndrome (IBS).

Dietician's notes

- This is a lovely moist chocolate cake, with only 4 g fat per slice. What a bargain! Please note that the cake should be cut into 20 pieces.
- Chocolate cake usually makes one constipated, because of all the refined ingredients and no fibre, but this chocolate cake should not have the same effect.
- It would be acceptable to have only salad and protein at your next meal, as you have already consumed your starch and fat at tea time.

Nutrients per slice
(using sugar)
Glycaemic Index 60 • Carbohydrates 23 g •
Protein 4 g • Fat 4 g • Fibre 1 g • kJ 617 •
Glycaemic load 14

ONE SLICE OF CAKE (USING SUGAR) IS EQUIVALENT TO
1½ STARCH + 1 FAT

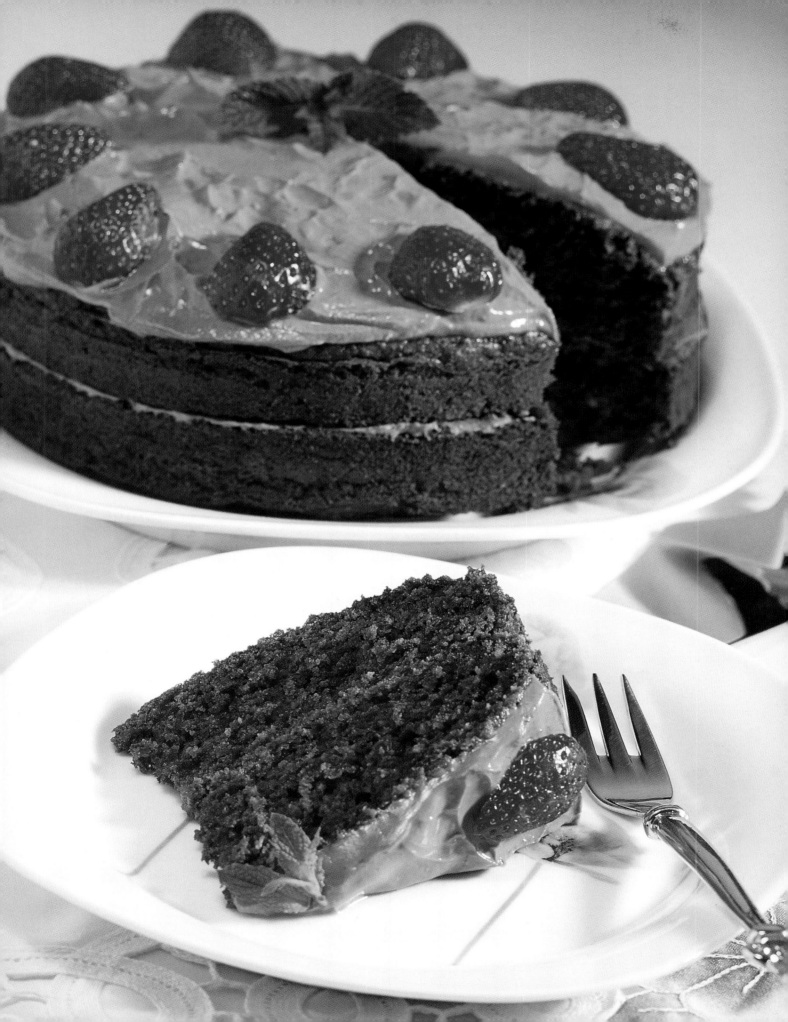

Hot cross buns

Makes 15

190 ml (¾ c) skimmed milk*, warmed slightly
150 ml (⅗ c) high-fibre cereal*
1 x 10 g sachet instant yeast
50 ml warm water
500 ml (2 c) cake flour
375 ml (1½ c) oat bran*
150 ml (⅗ c) whole-wheat ProNutro*
100 g soft lite margarine*
60 ml (4 T) soft brown sugar
80 ml (scant ⅓ c) mixed peel
190 ml (¾ c) sultanas
7 ml (1½ t) ground cinnamon
7 ml (1½ t) mixed spice
5 ml (1 t) salt
1 apple, very finely grated
1 egg, beaten
60 ml (4 T) cake flour

MIXTURE FOR THE CROSS
80 ml (scant ⅓ c) cake flour
60 ml (4 T) oat bran
80 ml (scant ⅓ c) skimmed milk

GLAZE
60 ml (4 T) skimmed milk

1   Pour ⅓ of the warmed skimmed milk onto the cereal, and set aside until soft. Sprinkle the yeast onto about 50 ml (⅕ c) warm water and leave until frothy.
2   Sift 500 ml (2 c) cake flour into a bowl. Mix the oat bran and ProNutro into the cake flour. Lift up a few times to incorporate air. Rub in the margarine until the mixture resembles breadcrumbs.
3   Add the sugar, fruit, cinnamon, mixed spice and salt to the flour mixture. Mix.
4   Add the apple, soft high-fibre cereal and frothy yeast. Mix.
5   Add the egg to the mixture. (Don't rinse the egg bowl; keep it for the glaze.)
6   Gradually add the remaining ⅔ of the milk to the mixture, as needed.
7   Add the extra flour, as needed.
8   Mix with a wooden spoon until the mixture forms a stiff dough.
9   Cover the bowl with clingwrap and stand in a warm place to prove the dough, i.e. until doubled in size.
10 Remove the dough from the bowl and punch down on a lightly floured surface.
11 Knead gently until the dough is soft and elastic.
12 Cut into 3 even-sized pieces, and cut these again into 5 pieces each, to make 15 even-sized balls.
13 Shape into buns, and place on a greased 18 cm x 28 cm baking sheet.
14 Cover with a warm, moist tea towel, and leave to rise in a warm place.
15 Preheat the oven to 200 °C.
16 Make the cross dough. Mix the flour, oat bran and milk until smooth.
17 Place in a plastic bag, cut off the corner and pipe a cross onto each bun.
18 Bake the buns for 15–20 minutes.
19 Make the glaze. Pour the skimmed milk into the bowl the egg was beaten in, and brush mixture over the warm hot cross buns.
20 Leave to cool before breaking the buns apart.

Microwave method

1   Prepare the dough and uncooked buns as described above.
2   Place 6 buns in a circle and microwave on high for 11–12 minutes.
3   Brush with the milk and place under a hot grill to brown the tops. Repeat for the remaining buns.

If the yeast does not froth up in the warm water, it has not been activated and must be discarded. You will need to get a new packet of yeast and use that instead.
  Hot cross buns also make a delicious breakfast at Easter time.

Dietician's notes

• It is important not to mix the batter too much as this improves digestibility which, in turn, increases the GI of the hot cross buns.
• Only use the quantity of flour called for in the recipe, as this is the ingredient that has the highest GI and will increase the GI of the buns if more is used.
• No commercial hot cross bun contains 5 g fibre!
• Even though we have halved the quantity of flour, replacing it with whole-wheat ProNutro, high-fibre cereal and oat bran, and we have used milk and low GI fruits, the GI is still 60! This is because the main ingredient of hot cross buns is flour.
• Please note the high Glycaemic load (GL). Eat only 1 hot cross bun with lower fat cheese as breakfast or a light meal or, if you have it for tea, remember to omit your starch at the next meal.

Nutrients per bun

Glycaemic Index 60 • Carbohydrates 32 g • Protein 6 g • Fat 5 g • Fibre 5 g • kJ 852 • Glycaemic load 19

ONE BUN IS EQUIVALENT TO
2 STARCH + 1 FAT

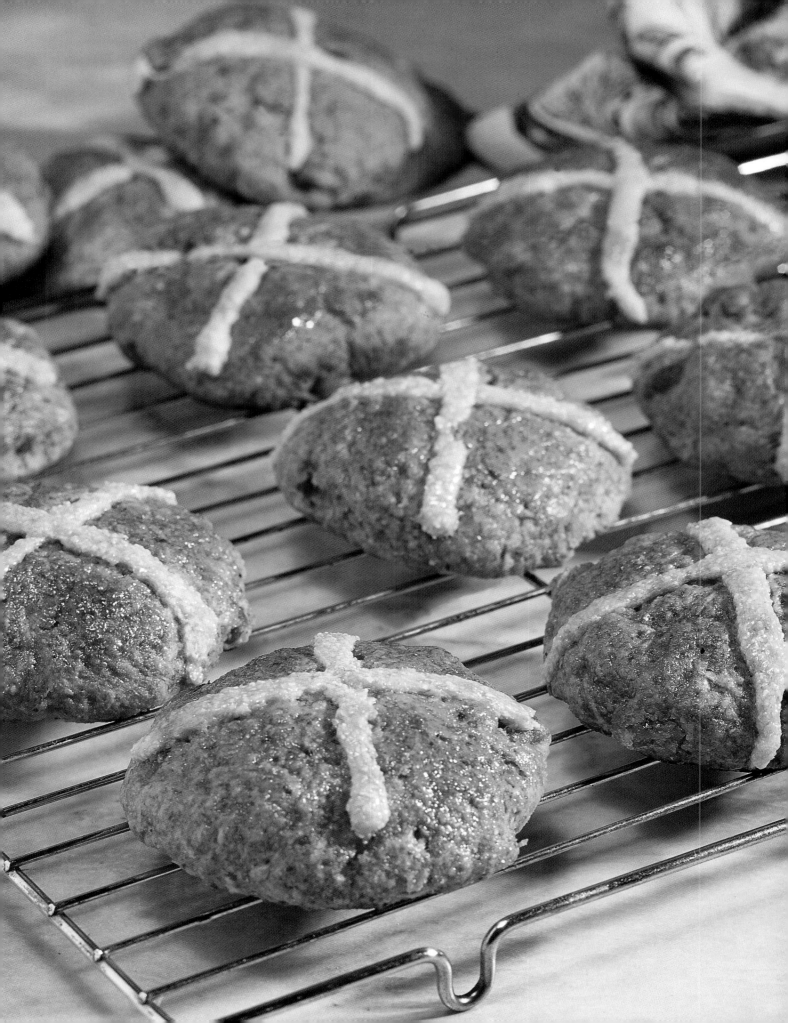

Chocolate brownies

Makes 15

1 x 410 g can white beans*, drained, or 250 ml (1 c) cooked dried white beans

60–80 ml (4 T to scant ⅓ c) skimmed milk*

250 ml (1 c) pie apples, unsweetened

15 ml (1 T) vanilla essence

200 ml (⅘ c) cake flour

10 ml (2 t) baking powder

2 ml (½ t) salt

125 ml (½ c) cocoa

2 eggs

1 egg white

250 ml (1 c) sugar

16 pecan or walnut halves, chopped

1 Preheat the oven to 180 °C.
2 Spray an 18 cm x 27 cm baking pan with nonstick spray.
3 Place the drained beans and half the milk in a food processor, liquidiser or blender, and process until smooth. Add more milk as needed.
4 Add the apples and vanilla essence, and process for 1 minute, until smooth.
5 Sift the flour, baking powder, salt and cocoa into a medium-sized bowl.
6 Beat the eggs and egg white in a large bowl. Add the sugar in 3 batches, beating for 1 minute after each addition, and using electric beaters.
7 Add a third of the bean and apple liquid mixture to the egg and sugar mixture, together with a third of the sifted dry ingredients. Fold in carefully. Repeat with the rest of the liquid and dry ingredients. Take care that all the 'wet' ingredients do not all sink to the bottom of the bowl. Fold in the chopped nuts.
8 Pour the batter into the greased baking pan and spread it out evenly.
9 Bake for 40–45 minutes, or until well risen. Before removing from the oven, insert a skewer into the centre of the cake. If it comes out with a little batter sticking to it, bake for another 10 minutes. If the skewer comes out clean, take it out of the oven and allow to cool for 5 minutes in the pan.
10 Cut into 15 squares (5 cm x 5 cm) and cool on a cooling rack.

These moist chocolate squares can be eaten on their own as a tea-time treat or straight from the oven as a pudding with chilled, whipped low-fat evaporated milk.

Dietician's note
- Any cooked or canned white beans can be used … butter beans, small white beans, cannellini beans or kidney beans.

Nutrients per brownie

Glycaemic Index 58 • Carbohydrates 24 g • Protein 4 g • Fat 3 g • Fibre 3 g • kJ 581 • Glycaemic load 14

ONE BROWNIE IS EQUIVALENT TO 1½ STARCH + ½ FAT

Buttermilk bran muffins

Makes 12

250 ml (1 c) digestive bran (wheat bran)

125 ml (½ c) oat bran*, pressed down

250 ml (1 c) low-fat buttermilk*

1 egg

125 ml (½ c) soft brown sugar

30 ml (2 T) oil*

5 ml (1 t) vanilla essence

125 ml (½ c) sultanas or low GI dried fruit, chopped

190 ml (¾ c) flour, sifted

5 ml (1 t) baking powder

5 ml (1 t) bicarbonate of soda

1 ml (¼ t) salt

1 apple, grated

1 Preheat the oven to 180 °C.
2 Mix the digestive bran, oat bran and buttermilk together, and set aside.
3 Beat the egg, sugar, oil and vanilla essence together.
4 Add the bran mixture to the egg mixture, and add the sultanas or dried fruit.
5 Sift the flour, baking powder, bicarbonate of soda and salt together, and fold the flour mixture and the grated apple into the batter.
6 Spoon into a lightly greased muffin pan, with 12 hollows.
7 Bake for 10 minutes, then increase the heat to 200 °C and bake for 5 minutes.

These muffins freeze well after baking.

For a moister muffin, leave the batter to stand for a few hours, or overnight, before cooking.

Dietician's notes
- If low-fat yoghurt (sweetened or unsweetened) is used instead of buttermilk, the GI goes down to 55.
- Adding a grated apple to any batter is a very effective way to reduce the GI value. Apples are also good at retaining moisture and adding sweetness, which means that, when an apple is used, the quantities of fat and sugar in the recipe can be reduced.

Nutrients per muffin

Glycaemic Index 58 • Carbohydrates 22 g • Protein 3 g • Fat 3 g • Fibre 3 g • kJ 548 • Glycaemic load 13

ONE MUFFIN IS EQUIVALENT TO 1 STARCH, 1 FRUIT + ½ FAT

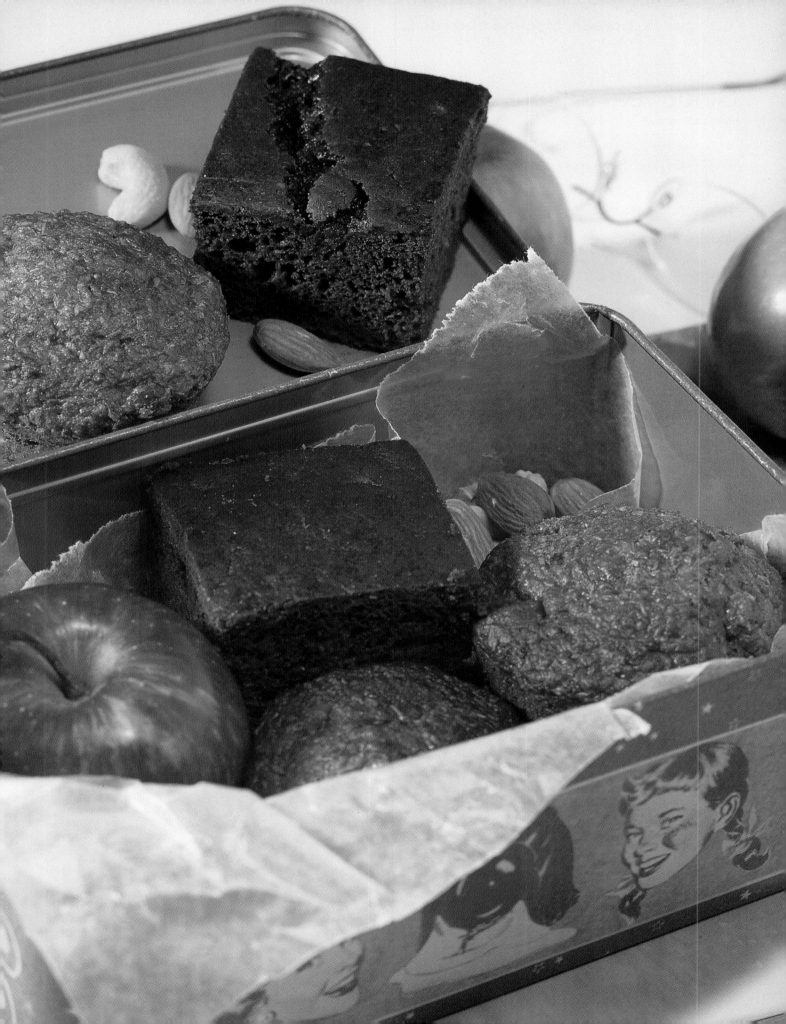

Ginger oat squares
Makes 15 squares

125 ml (½ c) cake flour
5 ml (1 t) bicarbonate of soda
5 ml (1 t) cream of tartar
60 ml (4 T) soft low-fat margarine*
75 ml (5 T) soft brown sugar or 90 ml (6 T) Sugalite
250 ml (1 c) oat bran*
125 ml (½ c) lower GI oats*
15 ml (1 T) ground ginger or 10 ml (2 t) chopped
  candied ginger
60 ml (4 T) fat-free plain yoghurt*

1 Preheat the oven to 180 °C.
2 Sift together the flour, bicarbonate of soda and cream of tartar. Set aside.
3 In another bowl, cream the soft margarine with the sugar and oat bran.
4 Add the oats, flour mixture and ginger, alternating with the yoghurt, and mix to form a stiff dough.
5 Spoon the dough into a greased 18 cm x 27 cm baking dish.
6 Dip your fingertips into some flour and gently press down the dough until the pan is evenly covered with cookie dough to a depth of about 5 mm.
7 Bake for 30 minutes, or until risen and golden brown.
8 Cut into 15 squares and cool in the dish.

Dietician's notes

* These ginger squares are ideal for those who prefer to leave out the starch and a little fat at dinner, in order to be able to have a sweet nibble afterwards.
* Because of their soluble fibre content, the high oat and oat bran content actively help to lower cholesterol levels.
* Even though there is 3 times as much lower GI oats and oat bran than high GI flour, the GI is still 60, which is close to the upper limit recommended for diabetics. This only shows how much impact flour, as ingredient, has on the GI of a food.
* For less chewy ginger squares, you could use Sugalite instead of the sugar. Use 90 ml (6 T) Sugalite in place of 75 ml (5 T) sugar. This will also lower the GI of the ginger squares as Sugalite contains polydextrose. See page 13–14 for more information on Sugalite and its constituents, polydextrose and lactitol.
* If you use Sugalite, do not eat more than 2 ginger oat squares at 1 sitting as 20 g of Sugalite has been known to cause cramping, flatulence and/or diarrhoea (1 ginger oat square contains 4 g Sugalite).
* Sugalite is not suitable for those suffering from Irritable Bowel Syndrome (IBS).

Nutrients per biscuit
Glycaemic Index 60 • Carbohydrates 12 g •
Protein 2 g • Fat 3 g • Fibre 2 g • kJ 343 •
Glycaemic load 7

ONE BISCUIT IS EQUIVALENT TO
½ STARCH + ½ FAT

Malawian sweet potato biscuits
Makes 20

200 ml (⅘ c) cooked sweet potato
  (250 g raw, with skin)
60 ml (4 T) soft 'lite' margarine*
60 ml (4 T) sugar
30 ml (2 T) fat-free milk*
190 ml (¾ cup) cake flour
10 ml (2 t) baking powder
1 ml (¼ t) salt
125 ml (½ c) oat bran*, pressed down
15 ml (1 T) castor sugar mixed with ground cinnamon

1 Preheat the oven to 180 °C.
2 Mash and cool the sweet potato slightly. In a bowl, mix the sweet potato with the margarine, sugar and milk.
3 Sift the flour, baking powder and salt over the sweet potato mixture, and stir to blend. Add the oat bran and mix to form a dough, using a wooden spoon.
4 Shape into a roll with a diameter of 4–5 cm; cover with clingwrap or waxed paper, and place in the freezer for 30 minutes.
5 Cut into 20 slices and place on a greased baking sheet.
6 Sprinkle with the cinnamon sugar and bake for 20–30 minutes, or until golden.

These biscuits are so delicious, you may want to double the recipe.

Dietician's notes

* Who would have thought that one could use sweet potato in biscuits? The sweet potato helps to lower the GI and makes the biscuits very moist.
* Although each biscuit contains about 5 ml (1 t) sugar, the soluble fibre from the sweet potato and the oat bran slows down the absorption of the sugar, making these biscuits suitable for those with diabetes.

Nutrients per biscuit
Glycaemic Index 62 • Carbohydrates 11 g •
Protein 1 g • Fat 2 g • Fibre 1 g • kJ 269 •
Glycaemic load 7

ONE BISCUIT IS EQUIVALENT TO
JUST UNDER ½ STARCH + ½ FAT

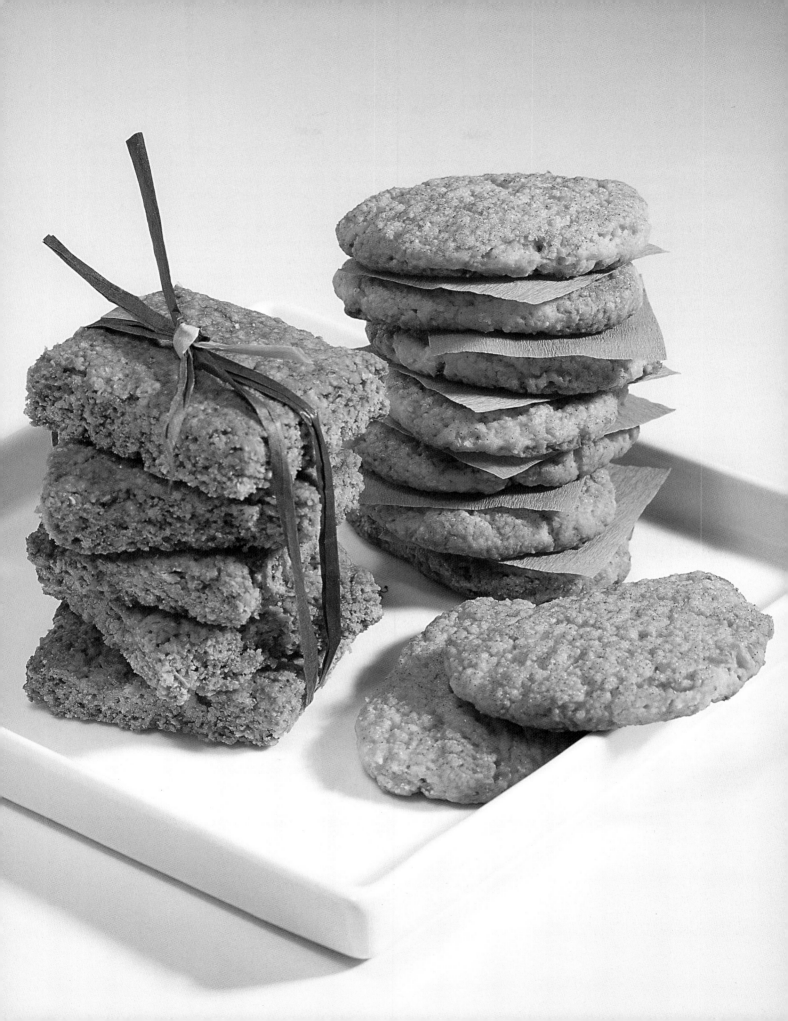

Nina's chocolate date squares

Makes 36 squares

125 ml (½ c) soft 'lite' margarine*

1 x 250 g packet dates, roughly chooped

1 x 410 g can butter beans*, blended, undrained,
    or 250 g cooked beans, blended with 50 ml (⅕ c)
    water

20 ml (4 t) vanilla essence

2–5 ml (½ to 1 t) rum or almond essence, depending
    on your preference

120 g nuts, chopped

500 ml (2 c) high-fibre cereal*

45 ml (3 T) cocoa powder

125 ml (½ c) soft brown sugar

100 g milk chocolate (does not have to be diabetic
    chocolate)

Nutrients per square

Glycaemic Index 54 • Carbohydrates 11 g •
Protein 2 g • Fat 4 g • Fibre 3 g • kJ 394 •
Glycaemic load 6

ONE CHOC-DATE SQUARE IS EQUIVALENT TO
½ STARCH + 1 FAT

---

1 Place the margarine and dates in a saucepan and gently heat until the margarine has melted. Add the pureéd butter beans and stir, breaking up the dates with a wooden spoon, to make a fairly smooth mixture.
2 Add the vanilla and rum or almond essence and chopped nuts, and boil for 2 minutes, stirring to mix well.
3 Add the cereal, cocoa powder and sugar to the mixture, and mix well.
4 Press the mixture into a 20 cm greased square or rectangular container.
5 Carefully melt the chocolate in the microwave or in a double boiler on the stove, and spread the chocolate smoothly over the date mixture.
6 Place the container in the fridge to set the mixture. Cut into 3.5 cm squares when the mixture has set, and store in an airtight container.

To make half the recipe, simply halve all the ingredients. The yield will then be 18–20 choc-date squares, depending on how you cut them.

Dietician's notes

- These rather moreish soft chocolate delights should be eaten only as a special treat, because of the higher fat content.
- Please note that 1 tiny square contains 4 g fat.
- These chocolate-date squares are meant to be a chocolate substitute. The GI of ordinary or plain chocolate is low, but the fat content is too high. These squares have less than half the fat of regular chocolate, a good fibre content and also a low GI and low GL. They're the perfect treat for those who suffer from diabetes.

Sultana and oat biscuits

Makes 40 biscuits

125 ml (½ c) soft 'lite' margarine*

125 ml (½ c) caramel brown sugar

125 ml (½ c) cake flour

1 ml (¼ t) salt

2 ml (½ t) bicarbonate of soda

5 ml (1 t) ground cinnamon

1 egg

500 ml (2 c) lower GI oats*

60 ml (4 T) whole-wheat ProNutro*

65 ml (¼ c) oat bran*, pressed down

250 ml (1 c) sultanas*

1 medium apple, cored, peeled and grated

Nutrients per biscuit

Glycemic Index 62 • Carbohydrates 10 g •
Protein 1 g • Fat 2 g • Fibre 1 g • kJ 277 •
Glycaemic load 6

ONE BISCUIT IS EQUIVALENT TO
½ STARCH + ½ FAT

---

1 Preheat the oven to 190 °C, and spray a baking sheet with nonstick spray.
2 Cream the margarine and sugar until fluffy.
3 In a separate bowl, sift the flour, salt, bicarbonate of soda and ground cinnamon together. Set aside.
4 Add the egg and a little of the dry ingredients to the margarine and sugar mixture, and mix well.
5 Add the oats, ProNutro, oat bran, sultanas and grated apple to the dry ingredients, and stir to coat all the fruit.
6 Add the dry ingredients to the margarine, sugar and egg mixture, and stir to make a stiff dough. Add some extra ProNutro or oat bran if the dough is too wet.
7 Spoon heaped teaspoonfuls of dough onto the greased baking sheet, about 5 cm apart, using 2 teaspoons. Bake for 15–20 minutes.
8 Lift the biscuits off the baking sheet, with a spatula, onto a cooling rack.

You will notice that it is rather difficult to mix this batter. Persevere and make sure all the sultanas are evenly mixed into the batter.

Dietician's note

- Eating 1 or 2 of these biscuits before exercise is ideal to ensure sustained energy levels during exercise lasting an hour or less.

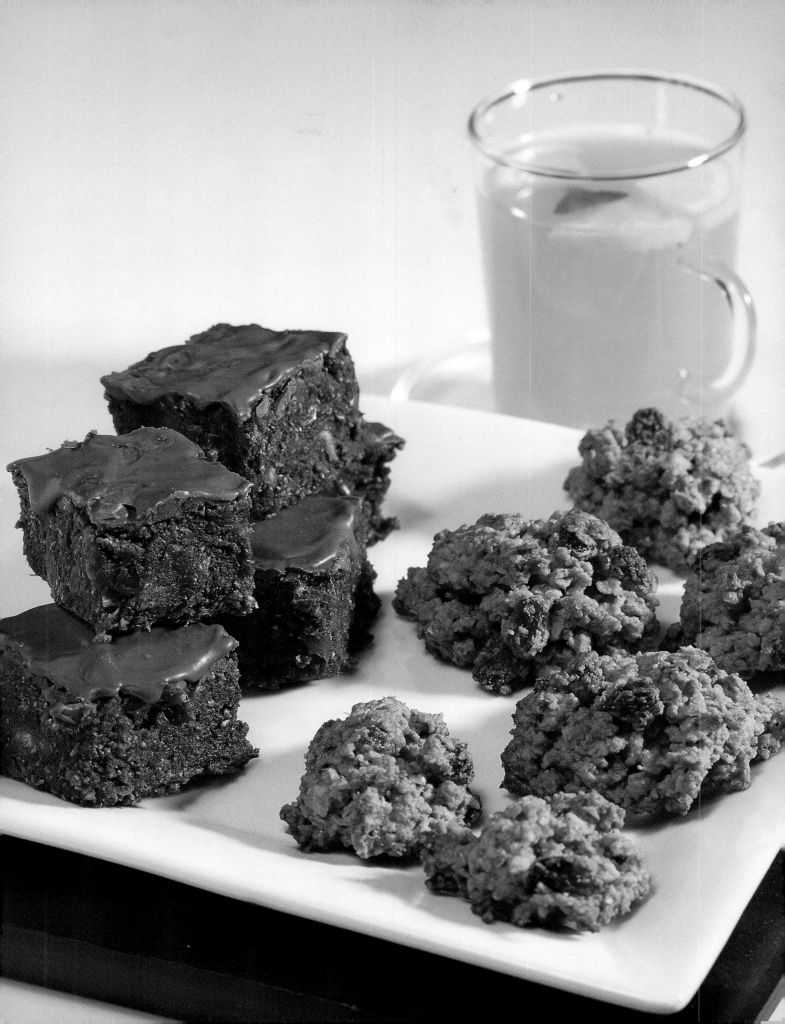

Rock cakes
Makes 25 biscuits

125 ml (½ c) soft 'lite' margarine*
80 ml (scant ⅓ c) soft brown sugar
1 egg, beaten
125 ml (½ c) cake flour, sifted
1 apple, peeled and grated
125 ml (½ c) sultanas
5 ml (1 t) baking powder
80 ml (scant ⅓ c) lower GI oats*
200 ml (⅘ c) whole-wheat ProNutro*
125 ml (½ c) high-fibre cereal*, crushed
2 ml (½ t) vanilla essence

Nutrients per biscuit
Glycaemic Index 57 • Carbohydrates 9 g •
Protein 2 g • Fat 3 g • Fibre 2 g • kJ 302 •
Glycaemic load 5

ONE BISCUIT IS EQUIVALENT TO
½ STARCH + ½ FAT

1 Preheat the oven to 180 °C.
2 Cream the margarine and sugar until light and creamy. Do not beat for longer than 2–3 minutes.
3 Lightly beat in the egg and 45 ml (3 T) of the flour.
4 Add the remainder of the flour to the margarine mixture, together with the apple, sultanas and the rest of the dry ingredients. Mix. Add the vanilla essence and mix.
5 Using 2 teaspoons, place heaps of batter onto a greased baking sheet.
6 Bake for 25–30 minutes.
7 Lift off the baking sheet while still warm, and cool on a wire cooling rack.

To crush the high-fibre cereal, pour it into a plastic bag and then crush it to the desired crumb size by rolling a rolling pin over the bag.

Dietician's note
- If raisins are used instead of sultanas, the GI will be slightly raised, to 59, because the GI of raisins is higher than that of sultanas.

Microwave health rusks
Makes 60 finger rusks

250 ml (1 c) lower GI oats*
500 ml (2 c) cake flour, sifted
25 ml (5 t) baking powder
5 ml (1 t) bicarbonate of soda
500 ml (2 c) digestive bran
500 ml (2 c) high-fibre cereal*
500 ml (2 c) whole-wheat ProNutro* (original or apple bake)
250 ml (1 c) sugar
5 ml (1 t) salt
250 ml (1 c) sultanas
2 apples, peeled and grated
100 ml (⅖ c) canola or olive oil*
1 litre (4 c) plain, fat-free yoghurt or fat-free fruit yoghurt*
250 ml (1 c) skimmed milk*
2 eggs
5 ml (1 t) vanilla essence

Nutrients per rusk
Glycaemic Index 52 • Carbohydrates 15 g •
Protein 3 g • Fat 2 g • Fibre 3 g • kJ 386 •
Glycaemic load 8

ONE RUSK IS EQUIVALENT TO
1 STARCH + ½ FAT

1 In a large bowl, mix all the dry ingredients together, using a wooden spoon to lift up the mixture a few times to incorporate air. Add the sultanas and the grated apples, and stir to mix.
2 In a large jug, mix together the oil, yoghurt, skimmed milk, eggs and vanilla essence. Add to the dry ingredients.
3 Mix the liquid ingredients with the dry ingredients until just blended.
4 Spoon the dough into 2 rectangular microwave dishes (e.g. Tupperware bread storer, 27 cm x 22 cm, or glass dishes of similar size) sprayed with nonstick spray and lined with paper towels.
5 Microwave each container on high for 18–20 minutes.
6 Check that the tops of the rusks are no longer moist when you remove them from the microwave oven. If they are still moist, microwave them for another 10 seconds at a time, until they are sealed on top.
7 Invert the baking pan onto a cooling rack. Carefully pull off the paper towel and leave the loaf to cool for 20 minutes before cutting into fingers. Cut into 30 fingers per bread pan, and then dry the rusks in a slow oven (100 °C for 2–3 hours).

This recipe can successfully be halved to make a smaller batch of rusks.

Dietician's notes
- The rusks are excellent as a pre-exercise, low GI meal or snack, because they help to lessen the blood glucose drop experienced after exercise.
- The low GI and low GL of these rusks makes them ideal snacks for diabetics, ADD children, and people suffering from hypoglycaemia.

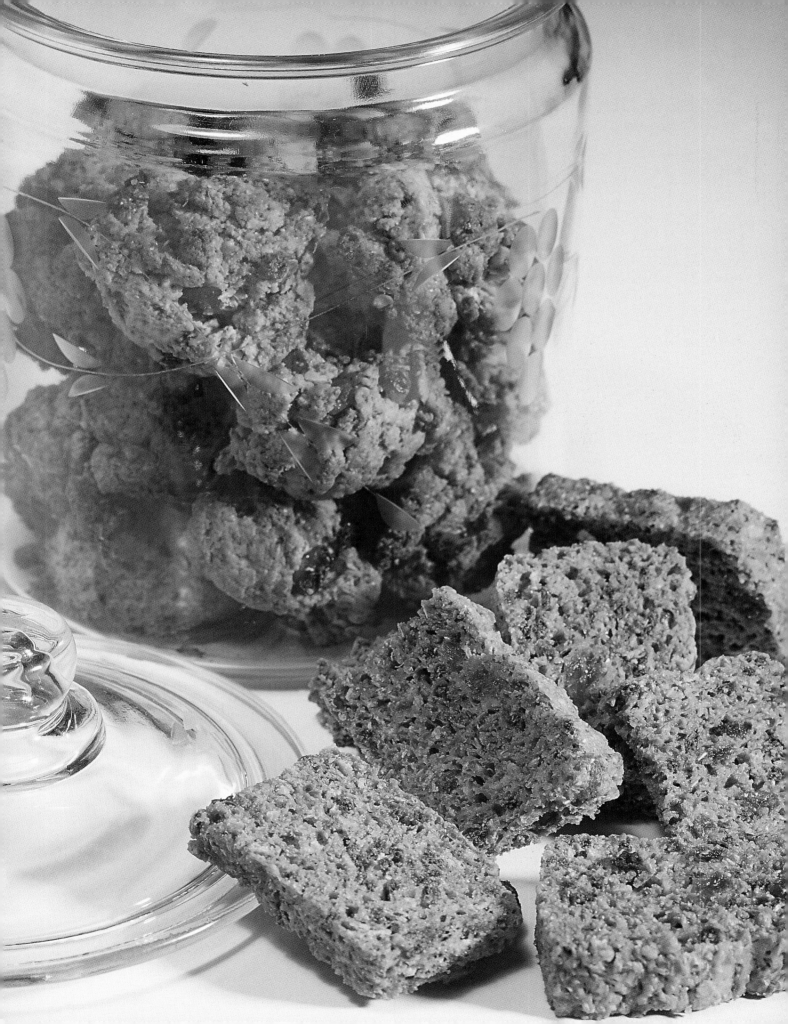

Jeske's buttermilk rusks

Makes 48 finger rusks

750 ml (3 c) cake flour

500 ml (2 c) oat bran*

250 ml (1 c) whole-wheat ProNutro* (original or apple bake flavour)

50 ml (⅕ c) baking powder

2 ml (½ t) salt

250 ml (1 c) white sugar or 375 ml (1½ c) Sugalite

125 ml (½ c) canola or macadamia oil*

500 ml (2 c) fat-free plain yoghurt*

2 eggs

2 small apples

5 ml (1 t) vanilla essence

5 ml (1 t) caramel essence

1 Preheat the oven to 170 °C.

2 Sift the flour into a very large bowl. Add the oat bran, ProNutro, baking powder, salt and sugar. Mix well, lifting the spoon to incorporate air.

3 In a 1 litre jug or bowl, measure off the oil, add the yoghurt and the eggs.

4 Mix well, until all the oil has been absorbed.

5 Peel and grate the apples. Add the apples and the vanilla and caramel essences to the yoghurt mixture and stir.

6 Pour the yoghurt mixture over the dry ingredients.

7 Stir well, until all the ingredients have been moistened to make a stiff, sticky, but spoonable dough.

8 Spoon into 2 greased 30 cm long bread pans, and smooth the surface.

9 Bake for 1 hour. Test the rusks with a skewer to make sure that they are done, before removing them from the oven. Bake for another 10 minutes if there is wet dough on the skewer when you pull it out.

10 When cooked, remove the pans from the oven, and leave to cool for half an hour or more. Then remove from the pans and cut into fingers.

11 Pack onto baking sheets and dry out in a low oven (50 °C) overnight.

12 Store in an airtight container.

These rusks have a little 'bran' in them from the ProNutro. If you prefer pure white rusks, leave out the ProNutro and use an extra 250 ml (1 c) oat bran in its place.

Dietitian's notes

- The GI will be lowered to 57 if you substitute 250 ml (1 c) of the flour with another 250 ml (1 c) whole-wheat ProNutro.
- Macadamia oil is a deliciously smooth and slightly sweet oil containing mainly beneficial monounsaturated fats … ideal for use in rusks.
- For a softer rusk, you could use Sugalite in place of the sugar. Use 250 g Sugalite in place of the sugar and reduce the oil to 85 ml (⅓ c). This will lower the GI and the fat content of the rusks, while improving the texture (see page 13–14 for a discussion of polydextrose and lactitol, the main constituents of Sugalite).
- Do not eat more than 2 rusks at one sitting, as more than 20 g Sugalite per portion has been known to cause cramps, flatulence and/or diarrhoea (1 rusk contains 5 g Sugalite).
- Sugalite is not suitable for those suffering from a spastic colon (Irritable Bowel Syndrome).

Nutrients per finger rusk

Glycaemic Index 59 • Carbohydrates 14 g • Protein 2 g • Fat 3 g • Fibre 2 g • kJ 402 • Glycaemic load 9

ONE RUSK IS EQUIVALENT TO 1 STARCH + ½ FAT

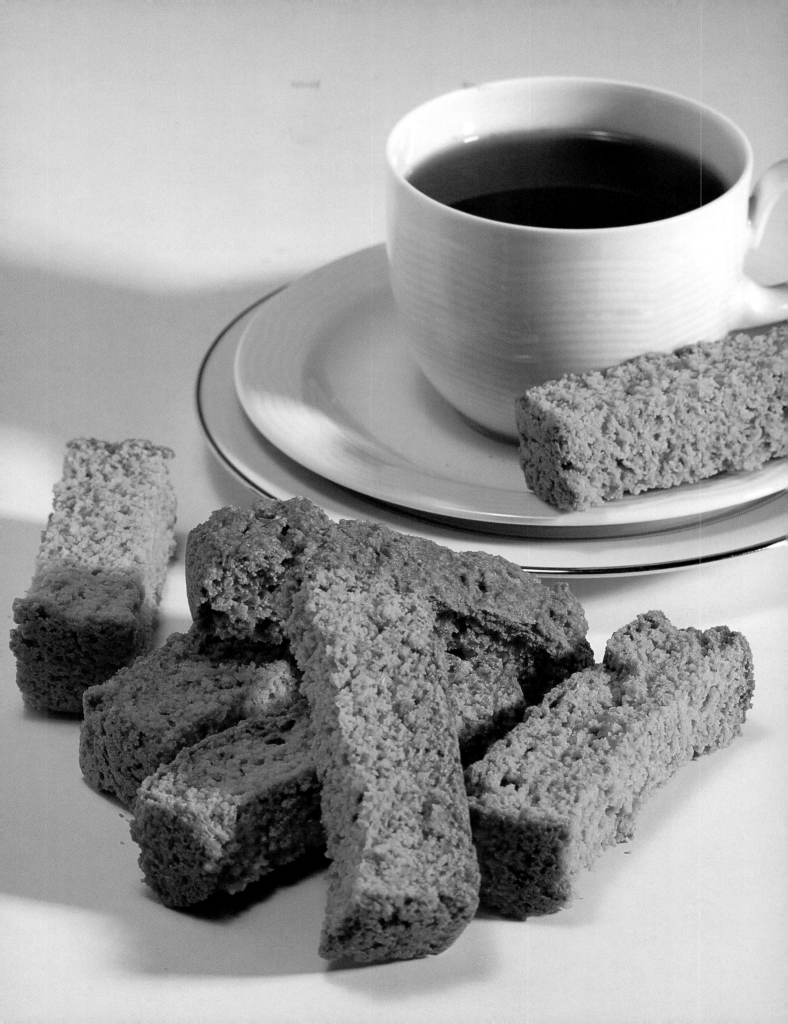

Honey and mustard dressing (Adapted from a recipe by Tabitha Hume)

Makes 200 ml (⅘ c)   Serves 10

60 ml (4 T) raw honey*
60 ml (4 T) balsamic vinegar
60 ml (4 T) whole-grain mustard

Nutrients per serving (20 ml = 4 t)
Glycaemic Index 55 • Carbohydrates 7 g •
Protein negl. • Fat negl. • KJ 137 • Fibre 0 g •
Glycaemic load 4

One serving (20 ml or 4 t) is equivalent to
½ starch

1 Heat the honey in a glass jar until runny (about 30 seconds on high in a microwave oven). Add the vinegar and mustard.
2 Stir vigorously in the jar until very thick. Spoon 20 ml (4 t) per person onto salad.

Dietician's notes

- The calculated GI of this dressing seems quite high because of the honey. However, the vinegar will bring the GI down in real life, so this is a wonderful, fat-free, low GI dressing.
- Remember, it is important to use raw honey as other honey has a higher GI.

Karla's creamy herb dressing

Makes about 300 ml (1⅕ c)   Serves 6

250 ml (1 c) fat-free plain yoghurt*
60 ml (4 T) 'lite' (lower fat) mayonnaise*
2 cloves garlic (less if you are not fond of garlic)
5 ml (1 t) finely chopped parsley
20 ml (4 t) fresh dill, finely chopped
    or 10 ml (2 T) dried dill
10–15 ml (2–3 t) sugar
3 grindings (2 ml [½ t]) black pepper

Nutrients per serving (50 ml = ⅕ c)
Glycaemic Index <40 • Carbohydrates 7 g •
Protein 3 g • Fat 1 g • Fibre negl • kJ 245 •
Glycaemic load 2

One serving (50 ml or ⅕ c) is equivalent to ½
dairy/milk

1 In a bowl, mix the yoghurt and mayonnaise.
2 Peel and chop up the garlic.
3 Add the garlic and herbs to the yoghurt mixture, then season with the sugar and pepper. Thin with skimmed milk, if too thick.

This salad dressing is best if served as a generous dollop of creamy dressing on a beautifully assembled salad.
    It is also delicious mixed with cucumber and served with a curry.

Dietician's notes

- This makes a deliciously rich dressing for any salad (even cold leftover cooked vegetables). The bonus is that it has a low fat content.
- People who have diabetes should note that the added sugar will have almost no effect on blood glucose levels because of the low GI, and the low GL.
- With the salad vegetables, the GL will not be more than 5, which means a salad with this tasty low-fat dressing will have very little effect on blood glucose levels. So enjoy to your heart's content!

Hummus

Makes 500 ml (2 c)   Serves 8

1 x 410 g can chickpeas* or 250 ml (1 c) cooked
    chickpeas
60 ml (4 T) lemon juice
5–10 ml (1–2 t) crushed or 1–2 cloves fresh garlic
60 ml (4 T) tahini (sesame seed paste)
salt, pepper, paprika, parsley

Nutrients per serving (65 ml = ¼ c)
Glycaemic Index <40 • Carbohydrates 8 g •
Protein 4 g • Fat 4 g • Fibre 2 g • kJ 348 •
Glycaemic load 2

One serving (65 ml or ¼ c) is equivalent to ½
starch and ½ protein, or 1 protein

1 Mix all the ingredients in a blender or food processor and season to taste.
2 Store in the fridge for up to 1 week.

This makes a delicious lower fat spread, in place of margarine or butter.
    Hummus is also delicious as a dip for vegetable crudités and pretzels, or as a side dish at a picnic.

Dietician's notes

- Peanut butter (30 ml [2 T]) can be used in place of the tahini.
- This bread spread is ideal for days when there is no time to prepare lunch; simply spread a generous quantity of the hummus onto a slice of bread, grab a piece of fruit and off you go.

Aubergine pâté

Makes 500 ml (2 c)   Serves 10

500 g (1 large or 3 medium-sized) aubergines (also
    called brinjals or eggplant)
15–20 ml (1–1½ T) lemon juice
4 cloves garlic, crushed
4 dried apricot halves, soaked in a little warm water
15 ml (1 T) peanut butter
2 ml (½ t) sesame oil
salt to taste
chilli powder to taste
65 ml (¼ c) plain fat-free yoghurt*
15 ml (1 T) chopped parsley
30 ml (2 T) chopped fresh coriander
5 ml (1 t) ground cumin

1 Preheat the oven to 180 °C.
2 Wash and prick the whole aubergines. Do not peel.
3 Bake in the oven until tender, 45-50 minutes, or microwave on high for 11minutes, until soft.
4 Allow to cool, then peel.
5 Place the aubergine flesh, lemon juice, garlic, softened apricots, peanut butter and sesame oil in a food processor and purée until smooth.
6 Remove from the food processor, season to taste with salt and chilli powder and stir in the yoghurt, parsley, coriander and cumin.

Serve as a snack or starter with lower GI crackers*.
This pâté also makes a lovely dip. Serve with vegetable crudités and low fat pretzels.

Dietician's note

*   This makes a perfect low GI, low-fat spread for low GI crackers and sandwiches. Used in such small quantities, it contains negligible kilojoules and has no effect on blood glucose levels.

Nutrients per serving (50 ml = ⅕ c)
Glycaemic Index <40 • Carbohydrate 3 g •
Protein 1 g • Fat 1 g • Fibre 1 g • kJ 115 •
Glycaemic load 1

ONE SERVING (50 ML OR ⅕ C) IS EQUIVALENT TO
1 LIMITED VEGETABLE

Mushroom sauce

Serves 4

1 x 250 g punnet mushrooms
½ medium onion, peeled
1 clove garlic
5 ml (1 t) canola or olive oil*
125 ml (½ c) skimmed milk*
5 ml (1 t) flour
5 ml (1 t) oat bran*
45 ml (3 T) water
2 ml (½ t) salt
freshly ground black pepper

1 Wipe mushrooms clean with a paper towel or wash them, if dirty.
2 Cut mushrooms in half or into thick slices.
3 Finely chop the onion and garlic.
4 Heat the oil in a frying pan until hot, then add the onion and garlic.
5 Fry gently over medium heat until the onions are transparent, about 5 minutes. Add the mushrooms and stir-fry for 2 minutes.
6 Pour the milk over; turn the heat down and simmer for 10 minutes.
7 Mix the flour and oat bran together in a cup. Add the water and mix to make a smooth, runny paste.
8 Pour the flour mixture into the milk and mushrooms, stirring all the time. Bring to the boil and cook until sauce is thickened, still stirring.
9 Season with salt and pepper.

Dietician's notes

*   Remember whenever you thicken a sauce, oat bran can be used in combination with the high GI flour to lower the GI, as we have done in this recipe.
*   This mushroom sauce can be used as a pasta sauce to serve 2 people. Cook 2 handfuls of pasta for 2 people and divide the sauce between them.
*   You can also add 100 g lean chopped ham to the pasta sauce. Add a mixed salad and you have a wonderful balanced meal.

Nutrients per serving
(sauce only)
Glycaemic Index <40 • Carbohydrates 6 g •
Protein 3 g • Fat 1 g • Fibre 1 g • kJ 202 •
Glycaemic load 1

ONE SERVING SAUCE IS EQUIVALENT TO
1 LIMITED VEGETABLE

ONE SERVING PASTA WITH HAM AND MUSHROOM
SAUCE IS EQUIVALENT TO 2 PROTEIN + 1 STARCH
+ 1 VEGETABLE

Party fruit punch

Makes 7 litres and serves 28 (without champagne) / Makes 7.75 litres and serves 31 (with champagne)

500 ml (2 c) pear juice*

500 ml (2 c) apple juice*

500 ml (2 c) apricot juice*

500 ml (2 c) orange juice*

500 ml (2 c) grapefruit juice*

5 ml (1 t) freshly grated ginger (optional)

2 x 410 g cans fruit salad* in fruit juice, drained

   or 500 ml (2 c) chopped mixed fresh low GI fruit

   e.g. apples, peaches, pears, apricots, plums,

   naartjies, berries or kiwi fruit

2 litres (8 c) diet lemonade or Sprite Zero*

2 litres (8 c) soda water

750 ml (1 bottle or 3 c) champagne (optional)

fresh mint for garnishing

1   Mix the fruit juices together.

2   Add the ginger, if using, and canned or fresh fruit, and chill well.

3   Add the cooled lemonade or Sprite Zero, soda water and champagne, if using, just before serving.

4   Garnish with the mint.

5   Ice cubes can be added.

Make the punch the day before, or the morning of your afternoon or evening party.

Dietician's notes

- What a delectable alternative to a regular fruit portion!
- Please note that any champagne can be used, as sweet champagne contains only 5 g sugar per glass, which will have a minimal effect on blood glucose levels. Dry champagne contains more alcohol than sweet champagne, and a little less sugar.
- The nutritional analysis was done using 125 g each of apples, apricots, peaches and strawberries. Any combination of low GI fruits should, however, yield a similar GI and GL.

See page 47 for a photograph of this recipe.

> **Nutrients per glass** (250 ml)
>
> Glycaemic Index 48 • Carbohydrates 12 g • Protein 0 • Fat 0 • Fibre 1 g • kJ 271 • Glycaemic load 6
>
> One glass (250 ml) is equivalent to 1 fruit

So where does alcohol fit in?

What many people don't realise is that alcohol can be viewed as a nutrient, just like protein, carbohydrate and fat. Yes, that's right! When consuming alcohol, therefore, remember the following:

- Alcohol contains kilojoules and therefore adds extra kilojoules to your daily intake, which can jeopardise weight loss and weight management.
- In addition, the human body prefers to use alcohol as an energy source, rather than fat. Consuming too much alcohol will therefore diminish fat loss, which it is important to note if you want to lose weight.
- It is better to have an alcoholic drink with a meal or a snack (such as the fruit and fruit juice in this punch), as alcohol is absorbed directly from the stomach and may cause hypoglycaemia if taken on an empty stomach.
- Consuming too much alcohol late at night can lead to high blood glucose levels in the morning, especially if you have diabetes. Always take alcohol in moderation, therefore, and always with food.
- Give preference to the following drinks, as they are lower in kilojoules and/or alcohol:

   Dry or 'lite' white wine

   Dry red wine

   Wine 'spritzer' (wine mixed with soda water)

   Dry sherry

   'Lite' beer

   Rock shandy, made with bitters and Sprite Zero

   Spirits such as whisky, brandy, vodka, etc. (Have a single tot and top it up again and again with soda water, caffeine-free diet cola or Sprite Zero.)

- If you are trying to maintain weight, do not consume more than 1–2 units of alcohol (if you are a woman) or 2–3 units (if you are a man). This is also a good guide for general health, as over-consumption of alcohol predisposes high blood pressure, high blood cholesterol levels, many types of cancer, osteoporosis, etc. Remember, however, that 1 unit of alcohol is equal to:

   125 ml (½ c) wine or champagne

   60 ml (4 T) sherry

   340 ml can or bottle 'lite' beer

   170 ml (½ x 340 ml can or bottle) regular beer

   25 ml (a single tot) of spirits

   250 ml (1 c) 'spritzer' (at least half should be soda water or ice)

   170 ml (½ x 340 ml can or bottle) apple cider

   80 ml (⅓ bottle) spirit coolers such as Smirnoff Spin.

Healthy breakfast smoothie

Serves 1

175 ml (1 small tub or ⅓ of a 500 ml tub) low-fat
  or fat-free plain yoghurt*
2 low GI fruits (e.g. apple, pear, orange, peach, kiwi
  fruit, plums, apricots) or 1 low GI plus
  1 Intermediate GI fruit (e.g. 1 small green banana,
  1 small mango)
5 pecan nuts, halved or 20 peanuts or 5 almonds
  or 5 cashews, chopped
5 ml (1 t) raw honey or soft brown sugar

1. Place the yoghurt in a blender.
2. Peel and chop the fruit. Add to the yoghurt in the blender.
3. Choose one of the nut types and add the required quantity.
4. Also add the honey or brown sugar.
5. Whiz around in the blender until smooth, but do not overmix.
6. Pour into a glass and enjoy your 'breakfast on the run'.

Dietician's notes

- Although a meal on the run is not ideal (and we certainly do not advocate it), this delicious smoothie will help to stave off hunger pangs for at least 4 hours.
- Remember not to make a habit of drinking smoothies instead of eating a balanced meal.
- Smoothies also make delicious desserts.
- Although this 'meal' does not seem to contain any starch, the sugar in the sweetened yoghurt, as well as the added sugar, make up a whole starch portion.
- If you look at the breakdown of this smoothie, it is the same as eating a regular breakfast – another reason why one should rather eat a regular, balanced breakfast than drink a 'milkshake'.

See page 24 for a photograph of this recipe.

Nutrients per serving

Glycaemic Index < 40 • Carbohydrates 53 g •
Protein 10 g • Fat 11 g • Fibre 5 g • kJ 1 430 •
Glycaemic load 19

ONE SERVING IS EQUIVALENT TO
2 FRUIT + 1 DAIRY + 1 STARCH + 1 FAT

Hot chocolate

Serves 1

125 ml (½ c) boiling water
10 ml (2 t) cocoa powder
10 ml (2 t) sugar or sweetener equivalent to 10 ml
  (2 t) sugar
65 ml (¼ cup) low-fat milk*
65 ml (¼ cup) skimmed milk*
2 ml (½ t) cocoa and sugar mixture

1. Pour the boiling water into a saucepan and dissolve the cocoa powder and sugar (if using) in it. Heat gently on the stove and add the low-fat milk.
2. When the mixture starts to bubble on top, stir continuously, using a whisk, until it boils, and then pour into a cup or mug.
3. If using sweetener instead of the sugar, add and stir.
4. Froth the skim milk in a milk frother or by using a milk frothing apparatus.
5. Pile onto the hot chocolate in the mug.
6. Sprinkle with the cocoa and sugar mixture.
7. Serve, and enjoy!

A cocoa and sugar mixure can be made by mixing 45 ml (3 T) cocoa with 75 ml (5 T) castor sugar in an old spice bottle, with holes in the lid.

Dietician's notes

- Skimmed milk makes the best froth, but if you want the creamier taste of low-fat or 2% milk, pour this into the bottom of the cup or saucepan and use the skimmed milk to make the froth only. A little vanilla essence can also be added to the skimmed milk in the milk frother, in order to improve the flavour of the froth on top of the hot chocolate.
- Please note that it is not recommended to use sugar in large quantities in drinks, as it affects blood glucose levels more markedly than when used in or with food. However, 10 ml (2 t) sugar can be used with safety in the hot chocolate, as the larger portion of milk should 'balance' out the sugar in the hot chocolate.

Nutrients per serving

Glycaemic Index 50 • Carbohydrates 15 g •
Protein 5 g • Fat 2 g • Fibre 0.5 g • kJ 416 •
Glycaemic load 8

ONE SERVING IS EQUIVALENT TO
1 DAIRY

Recommended food/product list

Lower Glycaemic Index and lower fat food products

Lower GI cereals and porridges

High-fibre cereals

Bokomo Fibre Plus
Bokomo Bran Flakes
Kellogg's Hi-Fibre Bran
Pick 'n Pay Choice Shredded Bran
Kellogg's Fruitful All Bran
ProNutro, whole-wheat, apple bake
ProNutro, whole-wheat, original

Lower GI oats

Bokomo Oats
Pick 'n Pay Choice Oats
Spar Oats
Woolworths Oats
Rolled oats
Jungle oat bran

Lower GI starches

Low GI pastas (durum wheat)
Fatti's & Moni's spaghetti and macaroni
Fatti's & Moni's pasta shapes
Fineform lasagne sheets and tagliatelle
Imported pastas
Woolworths dried pastas
Pick 'n Pay Choice pastas

Lower GI rice

Old Mill Stream brown rice
Tastic white rice
Tastic basmati rice
Veetee's basmati rice

Barley

Lion pearled barley
Crossbow pearled barley
Imbo pearled barley

Wheat rice/pearled wheat

Lion Stampkoring/Wheat Rice
Crossbow Stampkoring/pearled wheat

Lentils

Lion brown lentils
Crossbow whole lentils
Imbo whole lentils
Imbo split lentils
Lion split lentils
Crossbow split lentils
Tiger 4-in-1 Soup Mix

Dried beans, uncooked, and canned

All brands, and all varieties of dried
  beans:
All Gold
Crossbow
Farmgirl
Gold Crest
Gold Dish
Imbo
Koo
Lion
Marina
Mayfair
Pick 'n Pay Choice
Rhodes
Sunkist
Tiger 4-in-1 Soup Mix
Tiger split peas

Lower GI breads and crackers

Lower GI breads

Astoria rye breads, wheat free
Uncle Salie's homemade brown seed
  loaf
Old Cape Seed Loaf
Duens Seed Loaf
Woolworths Seed Loaf
Woolworths rye breads, wheat-free
Fine Form bread

Lower GI crackers

Provita, original
Provita, multigrain

Dairy products

Low-fat/fat-free fruit yoghurts (sweetened and unsweetened)

Clover Danone
Dairybelle
Parmalat
Gero
Pick 'n Pay Choice
Woolworths
Spar

Buttermilk

Parmalat, low fat
Dairybelle, low fat

Cheese

Lichten Blanc (Clover)
Dairybelle In Shape lower fat Cheddar
  (23% fat)
Elite Edam (24.5% fat)
Woolworths lower fat Cheddar
Woolworths lower fat Gouda
Mozzarella
Simonsberg Mozzarella (25.6% fat)

Low-fat, fat-free cottage cheese

(NB. Check labels for fat content)
Dairybelle
Lancewood
Parmalat
In Shape
Clover

Feta cheese

Pick 'n Pay Choice Danish Style
  (14% fat)
Simonsberg 33% reduced fat (18.7% fat)
Pick 'n Pay Choice Traditional (22% fat)
Clover Traditional (28.5% fat)
Simonsberg (29% fat)
Dairybelle Original (33% fat)

Ice cream

Dialite (all flavours)
Country Fresh Lite range
Mega Lite

Milk

Low-fat milk (2% fat)
Skimmed or fat-free milk
Nestlé Ideal low-fat evaporated milk
Parmalat low-fat buttermilk

Leaner meat choices

Ostrich

Klein Karoo ostrich meats
Woolworths ostrich meats

Bacon

Like-It-Lean bacon
Back bacon, fat trimmed off
Shoulder bacon, fat trimmed off

Minced meat

Extra-lean mince
Topside mince
Chicken mince
Veal mince

Tuna in brine

Pick 'n Pay Choice
John West
Gold Crest

Pilchards

Lucky Star
Glenryck
Pick 'n Pay Choice

Soya mince mixes

Imana
Vitamince
Veggie Mince

Lower fat mayonnaise and salad creams

Nola Lite reduced oil dressing (7.6% fat)
Trim low oil dressing (10.5% fat)
Weighless low oil dressing (10% fat)
Nola Slim-a-naise (12% fat)
Figure (12% fat)
Pick 'n Pay Choice low-oil salad cream
  (15% fat)
Kraft Miracle Whip Light (18% fat)
Crosse & Blackwell light mayonnaise
  (26% fat)
Hellmann's Light (31% fat)
Kraft Real Mayonnaise Light (34.6% fat)
Woolworths low-fat salad cream

Fruit juices

Grapefruit juice (fresh)
Ceres:
Apple
Cranberry and Kiwi
Secrets of the Valley
Mysteries of the Mountain
Orange
Whispers of Summer
Liqui-fruit:
Apple
Apricot
Breakfast Punch
Mango-orange
Passion Power
Peach-orange
Tangerine Teaser
Orange

Jam

Naturlite jams
Fine Form apricot jam
Weighless Strawberry jam
Raw honey

Oil

Olive oil, cold-pressed
Canola oil (Epic)
Macadamia oil
Red palm oil (Carotino)
Avocado oil
Peanut oil

Margarine

Flora light (50% fat)
Flora extra light (35% fat)
Flora liquid (78% fat)
Canola Lite (Blossom) (52% fat)

Lower fat coconut milk

Sunkist lite coconut milk
Taste of Thai lite coconut milk
Gold Crest lite coconut milk

Lower fat fruit and health bars

Trufruit dried fruit bars
Safari Just Fruit bars
Fine Form Green fig bar
PVM Zone bar
Bokomo Bran & Raisin bar

Please see the *South African Glycaemic Index Guide* by Gabi Steenkamp and Liesbet Delport, GIFSA 2003, for more detailed information on the GI of various foods eaten in South Africa (available from most bookstores, your dietician, or www.gifoundation.com)

Consult your dietician for help with lower GI lower fat food choices and meal plans.

For a list of dieticians in SA who use the GI in the treatment of patients, visit the website of the GI Foundation of SA (GIFSA) (see above).

For a general list of private-practicing dieticians in SA, visit the website of the Association for Dietetics in SA (ADSA) at www.dietetics.co.za

Index

alcohol 122
apricot sauce, Hake with 60
Aromatic fruit salad 86
Asparagus tart 46
Aubergine pâté 121
Aurelia's pizzas 38

baked pudding, Spicy 90
Banana bread 100
bars, Breakfast 24
bean bake, Corn and 64
Bean soup 32
Beef stew with green beans 78
berry pudding, Forest 90
Biltong quiche 38
biscuits, Malawian sweet potato 112
bobotie, Fish 58
bread, Banana 100
   Health 96
   Mealie 96
   Onion 98
Breakfast bars 24
Breakfast scones 24
broccoli casserole, Chicken and 48
brownies, Chocolate 110
Brussels sprouts with white sauce, Cauliflower and 76
buns, Hot cross 108
Buttermilk bran muffins 110
buttermilk rusks, Jeske's 118
Butternut soup 30
butternut, Roast sweet potatoes and 74
butternut, Stuffed 72

Cabbage stir-fry 68
Caramelised yoghurt and fruit 88
Cauliflower and Brussels sprouts with white sauce 76
cheesecake, Traditional German baked 102
chicken (kebabs), Satay 54
Chicken and broccoli casserole 48
chicken and vegetable curry, Thai 56
chicken casserole, Peachy 52
chicken mayonnaise, Cold curried 40
chicken, Mango 50
   Mustard 50
   Tandoori 52
   Unbelievable 48
Chilli con carne 78
Chocolate brownies 110
Chocolate cake 106
chocolate date squares, Nina's 114
chops, Chutney 80

Christmas fruit cake 104
Chutney chops 80
Cold curried chicken mayonnaise 40
Corn and bean bake 64
Cottage pie 80
Courgettes and mushrooms with white sauce 76
Creamy vegetable sauce for pasta 70
Crustless savoury tarts 46
   Asparagus 46
   Tuna and pineapple 46
Cucumber salad 34
curried chicken mayonnaise, Cold 40

date squares, Nina's chocolate 114
dressing, Honey and mustard 120
dressing, Karla's creamy herb 120

fish bake, Smoked 40
Fish bobotie 58
Fish pie 60
Forest berry pudding 90
Fridge tart 92
fritters, Sweetcorn 26
fruit cake, Christmas 104
fruit punch, Party 122
fruit salad, Aromatic 86

Ginger oat squares 112
Gingerbread 98
Glazed meatloaf (Microwave recipe) 82
Gooseberry fool 92
Gourmet green beans 72
Green bean relish (Kerrieboontjies) 36
green beans, Beef stew with 78
green beans, Gourmet 72

Hake mornay 58
Hake with apricot sauce 60
hake, Sweet and sour 62
Health bread 96
Healthy breakfast smoothie 123
Hearty winter soup 30
Honey and mustard dressing 120
Hot chocolate 123
Hot cross buns 108
Hummus 120

Jeske's buttermilk rusks 118

Karla's creamy herb dressing 120
Kerrieboontjies 36

lasagne, Lentil 66
lasagne, Tuna 62
lentil curry, Rice and 64
Lentil lasagne 66
lentil stew, Mushroom and 68

Macaroni cheese 42
Malawian sweet potato biscuits 112
Mango chicken 50
Mealie bread 96
meatloaf, Glazed (Microwave recipe) 82
Melktert (Milk tart) 94
Microwave health rusks 116
Milk tart 94
Mozarella herb muffins 26
muesli, Swiss 28
muffins, Buttermilk bran 110
    Mozarella herb 26
    Ursula's breakfast 28
Mushroom and lentil stew 68
Mushroom sauce 121
mushrooms with white sauce, Courgettes and 76
Mustard chicken 50

Napolitana sauce for pasta 70
Nina's chocolate date squares 114

oat biscuits, Sultana and 114
oat squares, Ginger 112
Onion bread 98
Ostrich bourguignonne 84
    Variation: Venison pie 84

Pancakes 42
Party fruit punch 122
pasta sauce, Creamy vegetable 70
pasta sauce, Napolitana 70
pâté, Aubergine 121
Peachy chicken casserole 52
peanut sauce (satay sauce) 54
pie, Fish 60
Pineapple fluff 86
pizzas, Aurelia's 38

quiche, Biltong 38
quiche, Tomato and onion 44
Quick ['n] easy minestrone soup 32

relish, Green bean (Kerrieboontjies) 36
Rice and lentil curry 64
Roast sweet potatoes and butternut 74
Roast vegetables 74
Rock cakes 116
rusks, Jeske's buttermilk 118

Microwave health 116
salad with pears, Waldorf 36
salad, Cucumber 34
'salad', Winter 34
Satay chicken (kebabs) 54
sauce, Mushroom 121
    satay (peanut butter) 54
scones, Breakfast 24
Smoked fish bake 40
smoothie, Healthy breakfast 123
soup, Bean 32
    Butternut 30
    Hearty winter 30
    minestrone, Quick ['n] easy 32
    Winter 'salad' 34
Spaghetti bolognaise 82
Spicy baked pudding 90
stir-fry, Cabbage 68
Stuffed butternut 72
Sultana and oat biscuits 114
Sweet and sour hake 62
sweet potato biscuits, Malawian 112
sweet potatoes and butternut, Roast 74
Sweetcorn fritters 26
Swiss muesli 28

Tandoori chicken 52
tart, Crustless Asparagus 46
    Crustless Tuna and pineapple 46
    Fridge 92
    Tipsy 88
Thai chicken and vegetable curry 56
Tipsy tart 88
Tomato and onion quiche 44
Traditional German baked cheesecake 102
Tuna and pineapple tart 46
Tuna lasagne 62

Unbelievable chicken 48
Ursula's breakfast muffins 28

vegetable curry, Thai chicken and 56
Vegetable duos with white sauce 76
    Cauliflower and Brussels sprouts 76
    Courgettes and mushrooms 76
vegetable sauce, creamy, for pasta 70
vegetables, Roast 74
Venison pie (Variation: Ostrich bourguignonne) 84

Waldorf salad with pears 36
white sauce 76
Winter 'salad' 34

yoghurt and fruit, Caramelised 88

Acknowledgements

A great big thank you to our families, for their patience and support while we prepared
and tried out all these dishes over and over again until they were perfect, and for the many family
hours they gave up to get this cookery book completed.
Thank you also to Engela van Eyssen from the Dry Bean Producers Organisation for her assistance with the food
styling, and to Willie van Heerden for his professional, yet fun, input with the photographs.
To my dear friend Ursula, who embraced the lower GI, lower fat concept with enthusiasm,
and developed several wonderful recipes for this book.
To Jeske Wellmann RD(SA) for her cheerful willingness to help with recipe analysis, even at short notice.
To Anne, Sue and Linda, our secretaries, who worked for many hours to finalise the document for publishing.
To all our colleagues, for their support of this project and for their enthusiastic
use of our first recipe book for their patients.
To Tony Burdzik, of Harrie's Pancakes, for his generous hospitality and invaluable
input while finalising the recipes. His flair and experience as a chef inspired us to more creativity
in putting the finishing touches to the dishes.
We also humbly acknowledge the hand of the Lord in bringing this book to fruition.